My Degeneration

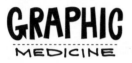

SUSAN MERRILL SQUIER AND IAN WILLIAMS, GENERAL EDITORS

EDITORIAL COLLECTIVE

MK Czerwiec (Northwestern University)

Michael J. Green (Penn State University College of Medicine)

Kimberly R. Myers (Penn State University College of Medicine)

Scott T. Smith (Penn State University)

OTHER TITLES IN THE SERIES:

MK Czerwiec, Ian Williams, Susan Merrill Squier, Michael J. Green, Kimberly R. Myers, and Scott T. Smith, *Graphic Medicine Manifesto*

Ian Williams, *The Bad Doctor: The Troubled Life and Times of Dr. Iwan James*

Books in the Graphic Medicine series are inspired by a growing awareness of the value of comics as an important resource for communicating about a range of issues broadly termed "medical." For healthcare practitioners, patients, families, and caregivers dealing with illness and disability, graphic narrative enlightens complicated or difficult experience. For scholars in literary, cultural, and comics studies, the genre articulates a complex and powerful analysis of illness, medicine, and disability and a rethinking of the boundaries of "health." The series includes original comics from artists and non-artists alike, such as self-reflective "graphic pathographies" or comics used in medical training and education, as well as monographic studies and edited collections from scholars, practitioners, and medical educators.

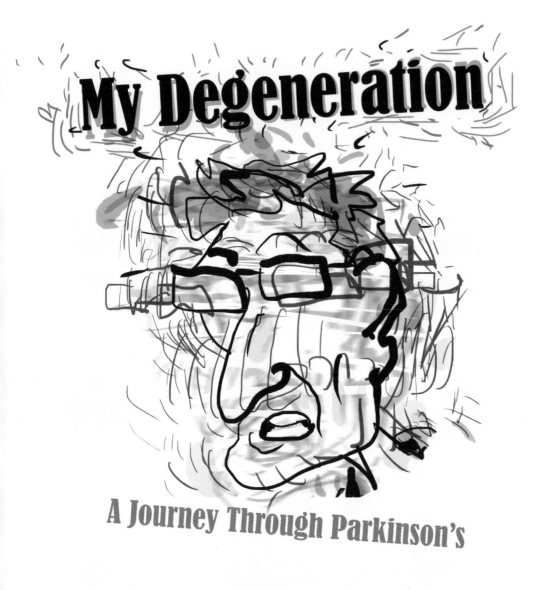

My Degeneration

A Journey Through Parkinson's

Peter Dunlap-Shohl

The Pennsylvania State University Press | University Park, Pennsylvania

Library of Congress Cataloging-in-
Publication Data

Dunlap-Shohl, Peter, 1958– , author, book
artist
My degeneration : a journey through
Parkinson's / Peter Dunlap-Shohl.
        p.   cm.
Summary: "A narrative of the author's
battle with Parkinson's disease. Traces
the author's journey through depression,
the disease symptoms, the medication
and its side effects, the author's
interactions with family, and the mental
and physical changes caused by the
disease"—Provided by publisher.
ISBN 978-0-271-07102-2
(pbk. : alk. paper)
I. Title.
[DNLM: 1. Dunlap-Shohl, Peter, 1958– .
2. Parkinson Disease—psychology—
Cartoons. 3. Parkinson Disease—
psychology—Personal Narratives.
4. Parkinson Disease—diagnosis—
Cartoons. 5. Parkinson Disease—
diagnosis—Personal Narratives.
6. Parkinson Disease—drug therapy—
Cartoons. 7. Parkinson Disease—drug
therapy—Personal Narratives. WL 359]
RC382
616.8'33—dc23
2015020290

Printed in Hong Kong by
Regent Publishing Services
Published by
The Pennsylvania State University Press,
University Park, PA 16802–1003

0 9 8 7 6 5 4 3

The Pennsylvania State University Press is
a member of the Association of American
University Presses.

It is the policy of The Pennsylvania State
University Press to use acid-free paper.
Publications on uncoated stock satisfy
the minimum requirements of American
National Standard for Information
Sciences—Permanence of Paper for
Printed Library Material,
ANSI Z39.48–1992.

To Pamela Dunlap-Shohl, my wife

Contents

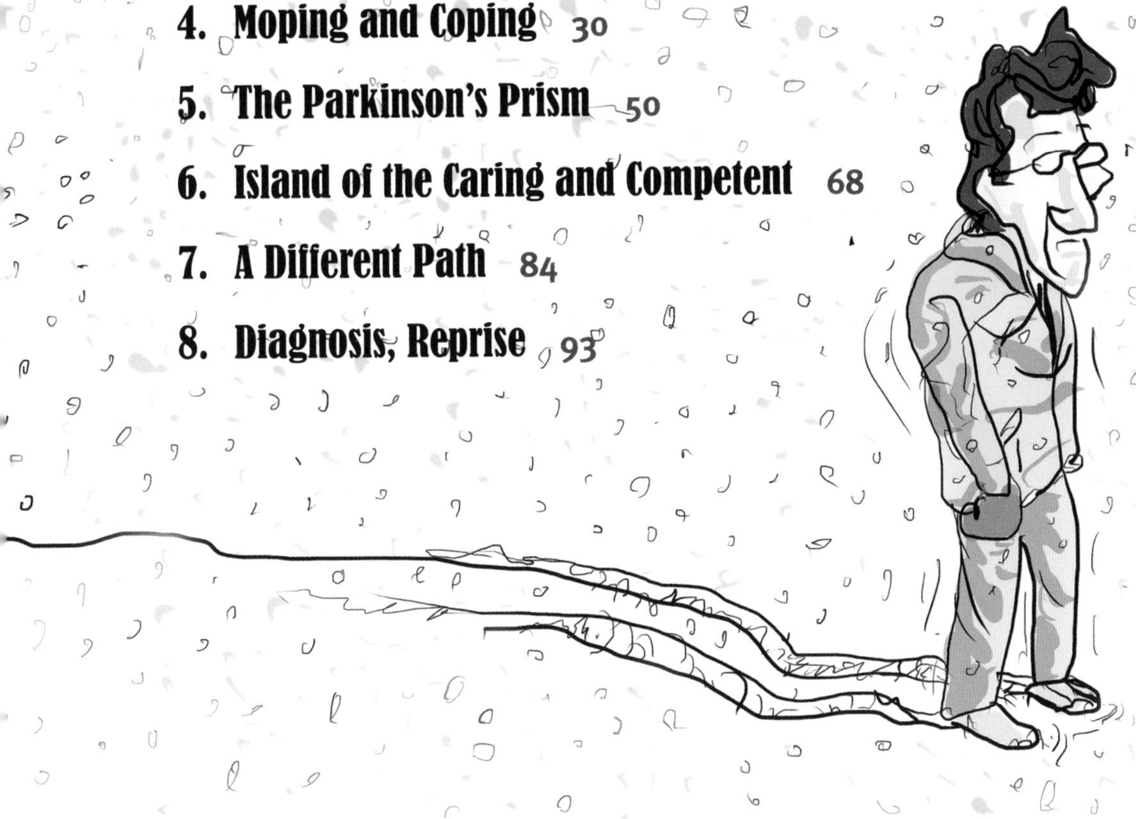

Acknowledgments

This work would not exist if Steve Aufrecht hadn't convinced me that I had something different to add to the mass of existing accounts of struggles with Parkinson's Disease. It would be far more difficult to follow without the guidance of Kendra Boileau and others at Penn State Press. It would have been less informative without the generosity and research of Dr. David Heydrick. It would be markedly clumsier without the patient suggestions of my sister Margo Shohl Rosen, and it would be unthinkable without the stalwart love of my wife, Pamela Dunlap-Shohl, to whom it is dedicated.

1. Diagnosis Blues

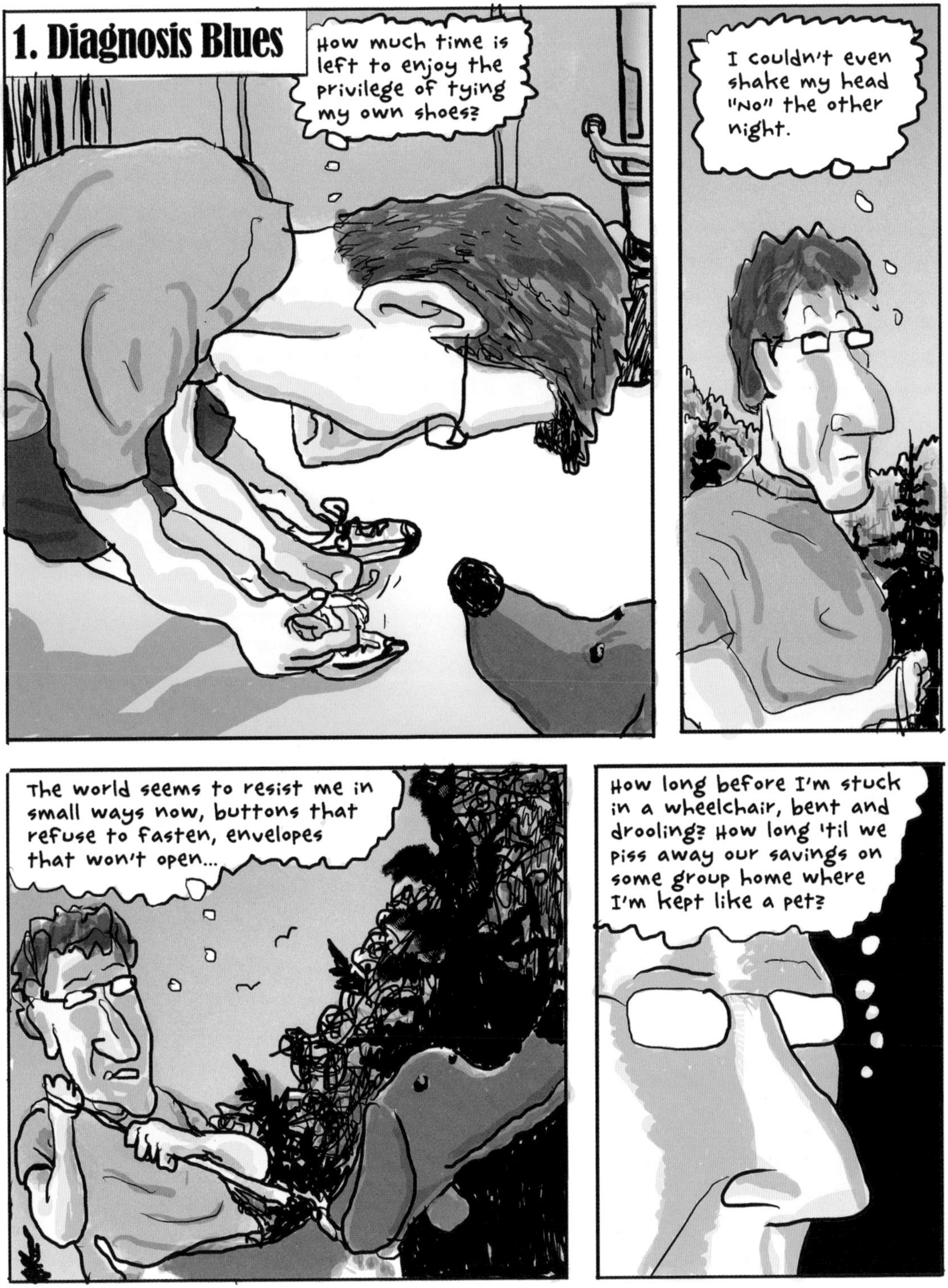
How much time is left to enjoy the privilege of tying my own shoes?
I couldn't even shake my head "No" the other night.
The world seems to resist me in small ways now, buttons that refuse to fasten, envelopes that won't open...
How long before I'm stuck in a wheelchair, bent and drooling? How long 'til we piss away our savings on some group home where I'm kept like a pet?

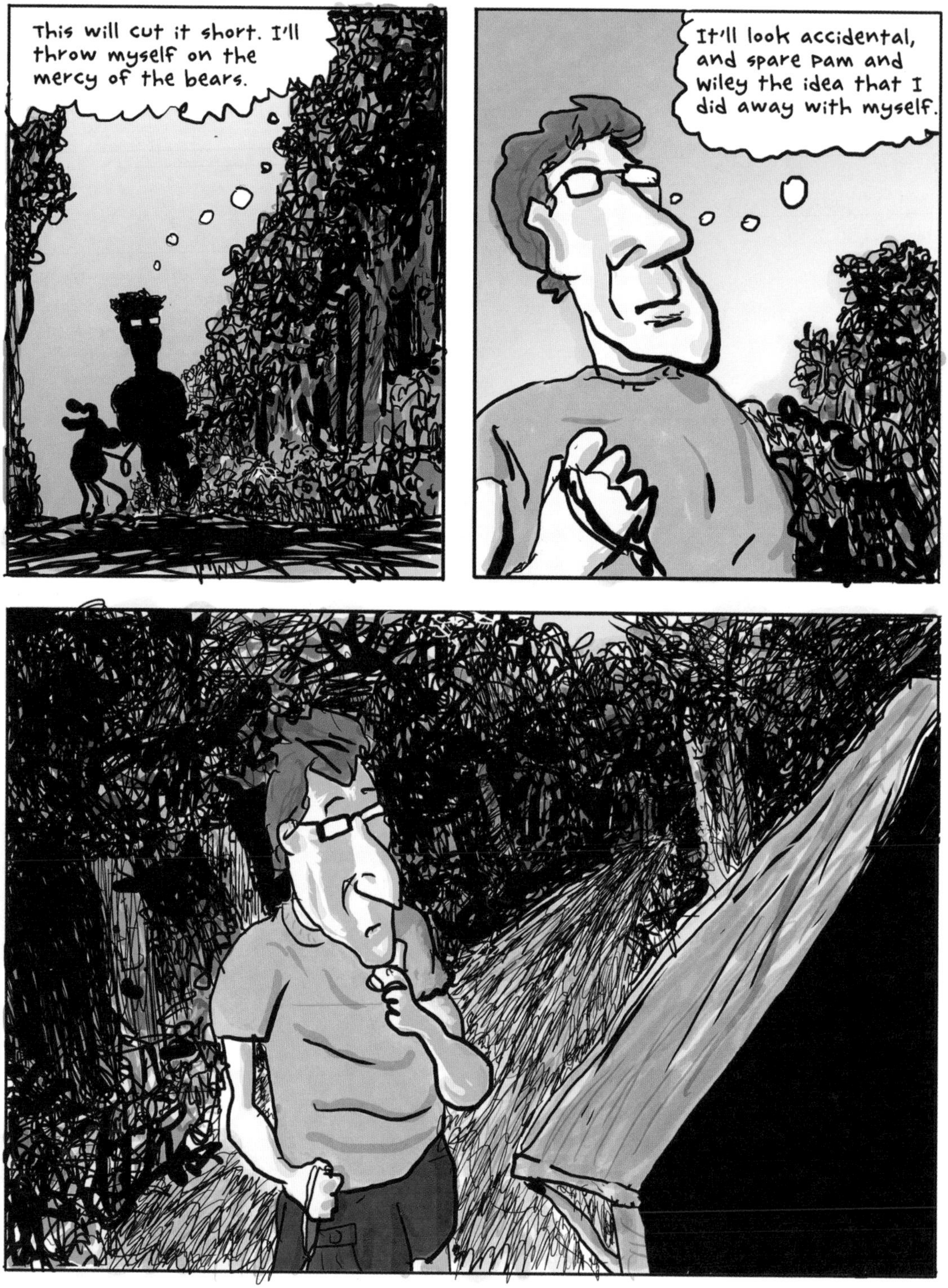
This will cut it short. I'll throw myself on the mercy of the bears.
It'll look accidental, and spare Pam and Wiley the idea that I did away with myself.

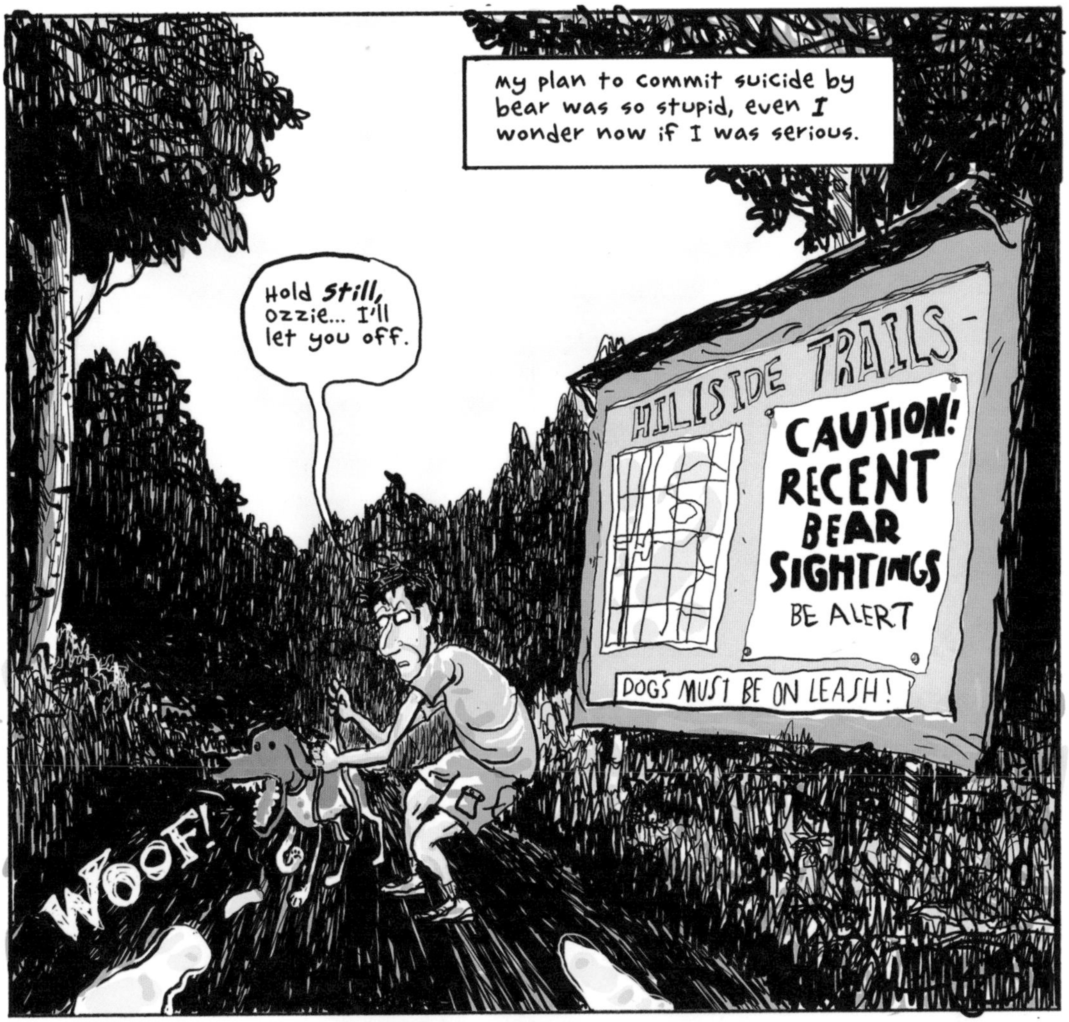
My plan to commit suicide by bear was so stupid, even *I* wonder now if I was serious.
Hold *Still*, ozzie... I'll let you off.
HILLSIDE TRAILS
CAUTION! RECENT BEAR SIGHTINGS
BE ALERT
DOGS MUST BE ON LEASH!
WOOF!

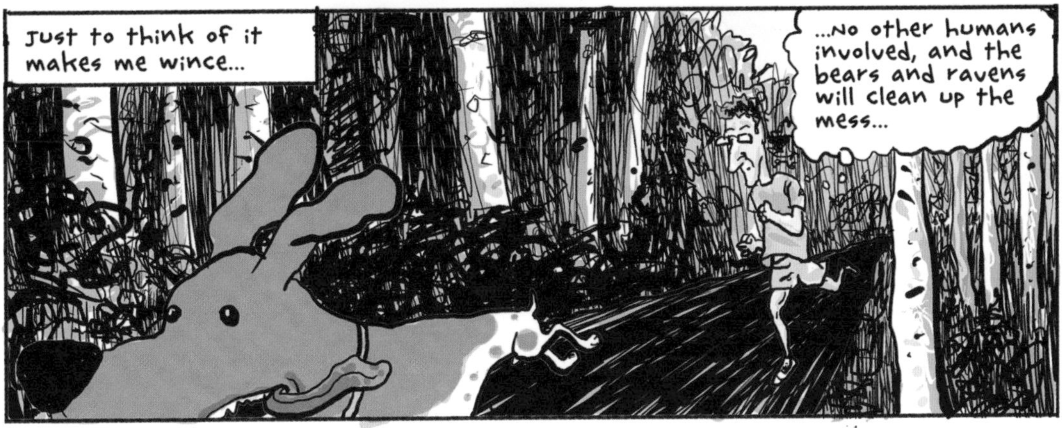
Just to think of it makes me wince...
...No other humans involved, and the bears and ravens will clean up the mess...

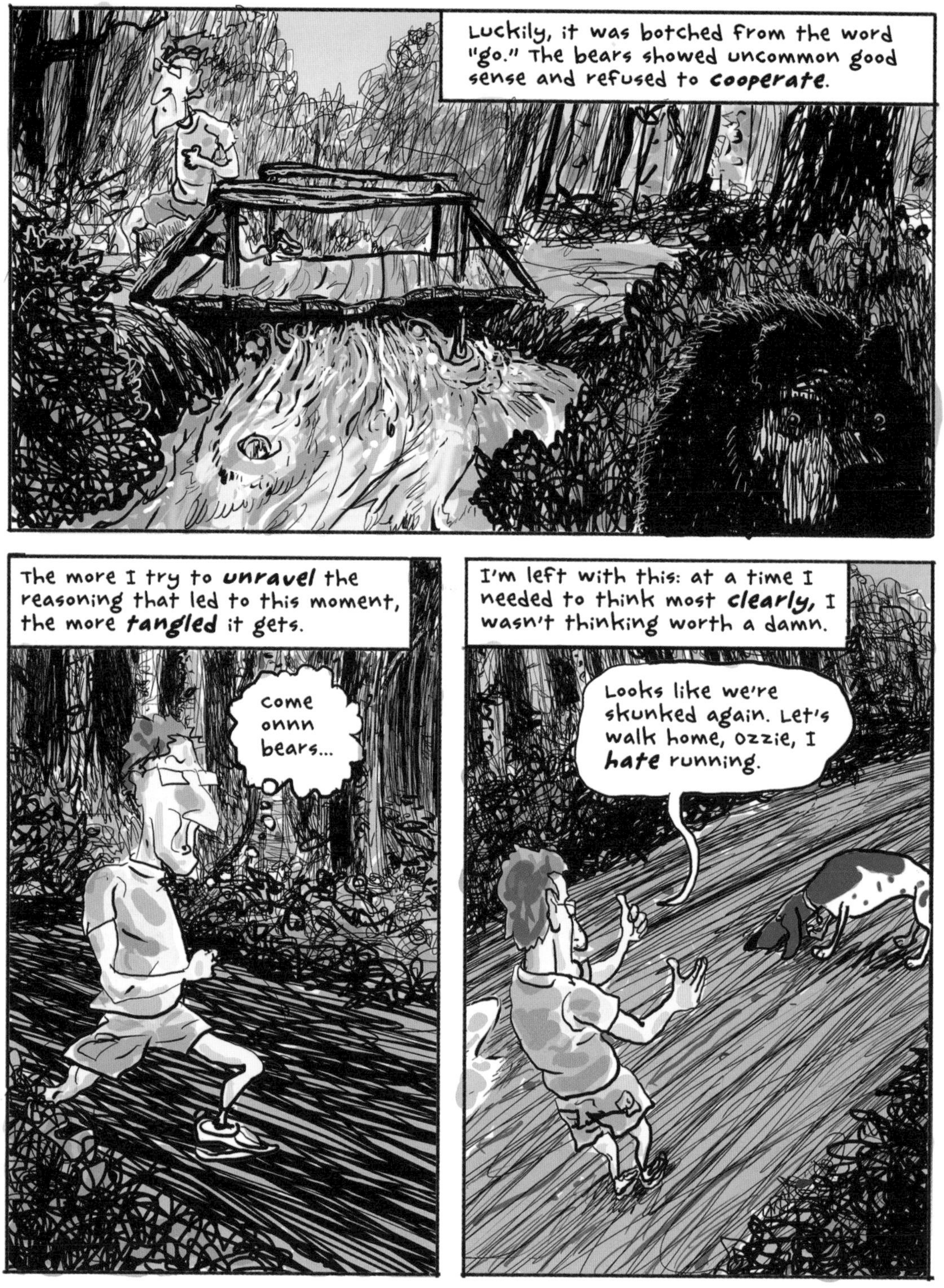
Luckily, it was botched from the word "go." The bears showed uncommon good sense and refused to *cooperate*.
The more I try to *unravel* the reasoning that led to this moment, the more *tangled* it gets.
come onnn bears...
I'm left with this: at a time I needed to think most *clearly*, I wasn't thinking worth a damn.
Looks like we're skunked again. Let's walk home, Ozzie, I *hate* running.

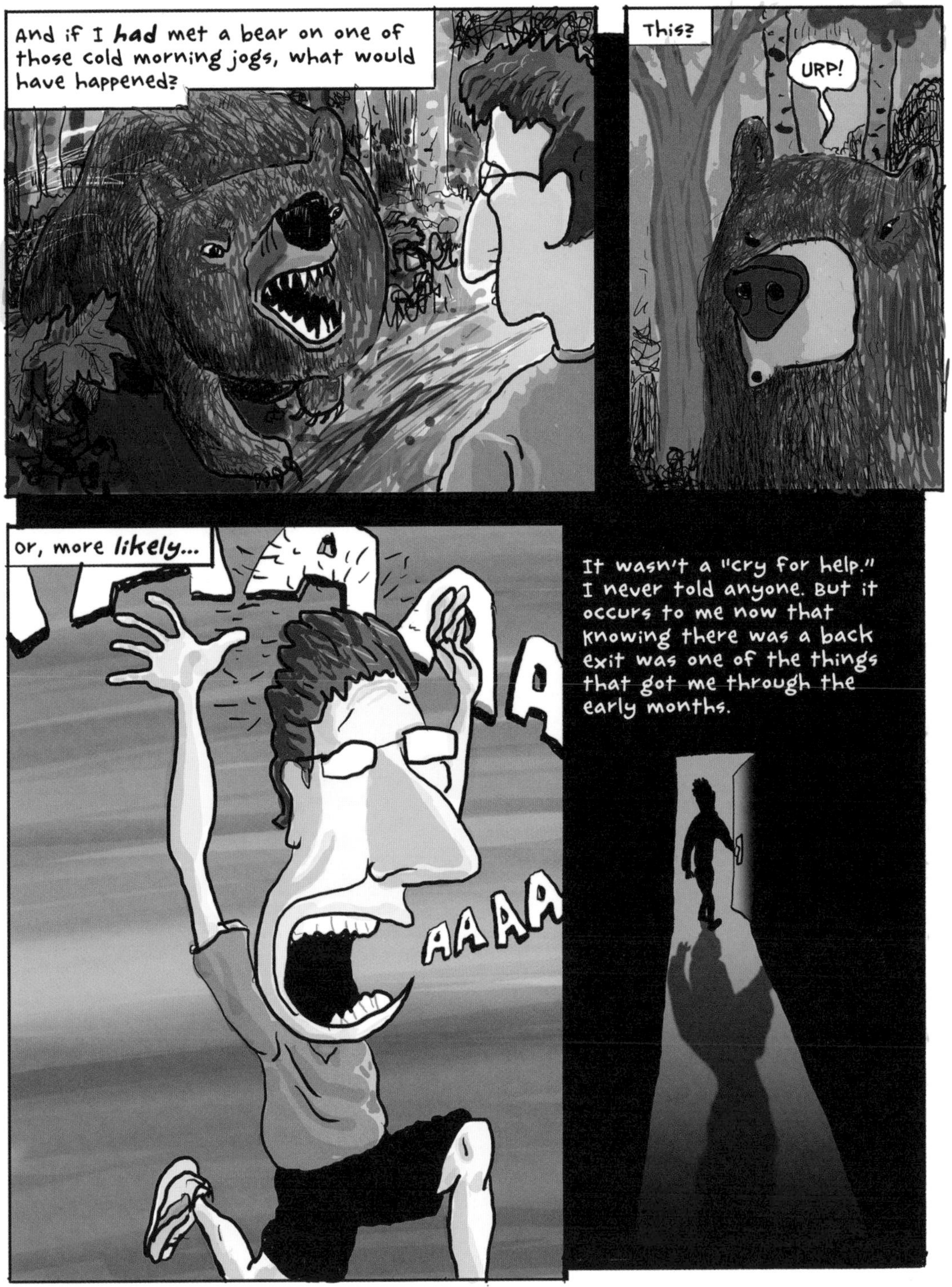
And if I **had** met a bear on one of those cold morning jogs, what would have happened?
This?
URP!
or, more **likely**...
AAAAA
It wasn't a "cry for help." I never told anyone. But it occurs to me now that knowing there was a back exit was one of the things that got me through the early months.

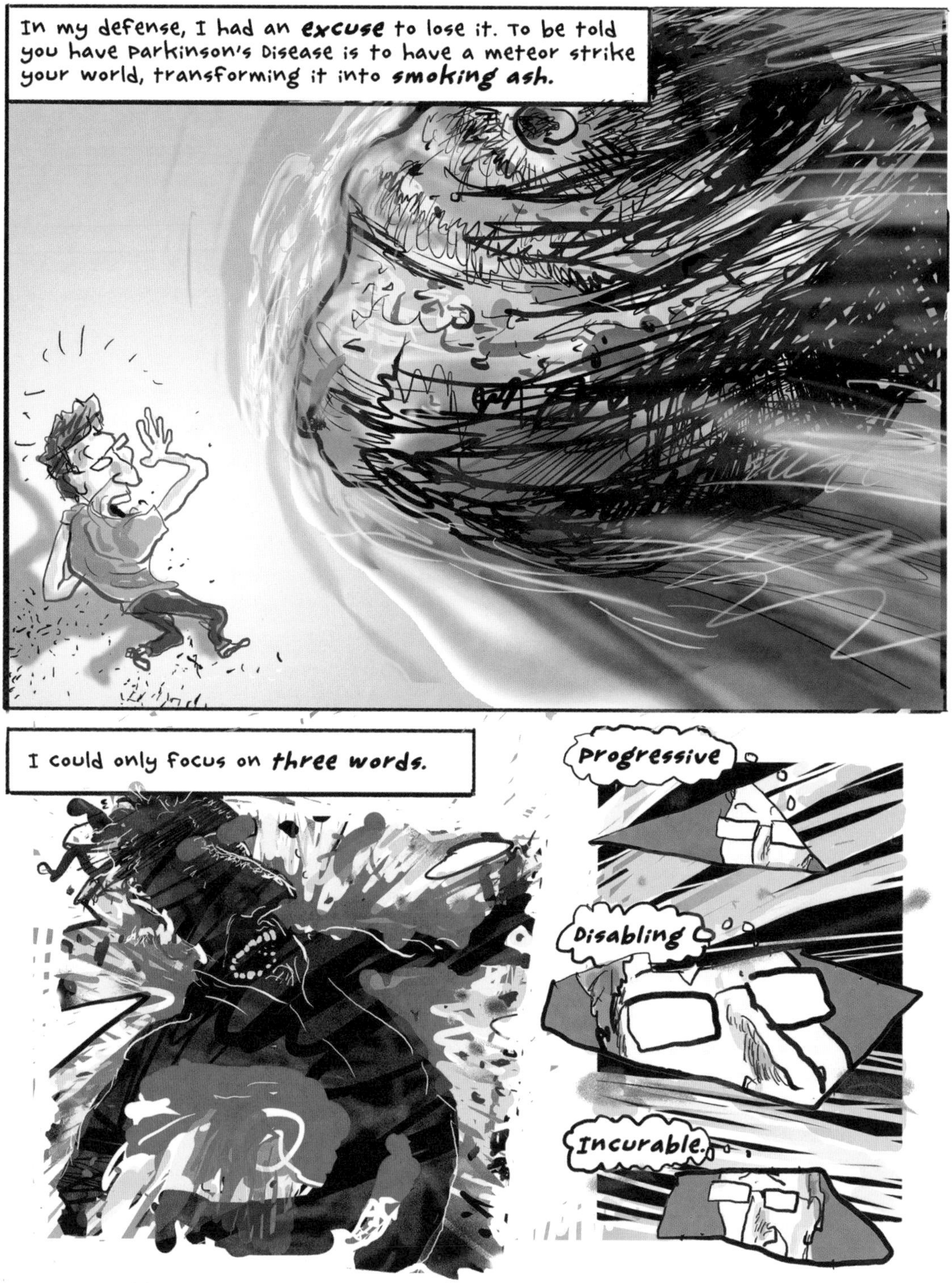
In my defense, I had an *excuse* to lose it. To be told you have Parkinson's Disease is to have a meteor strike your world, transforming it into *smoking ash.*
I could only focus on *three words.*
Progressive
Disabling
Incurable.

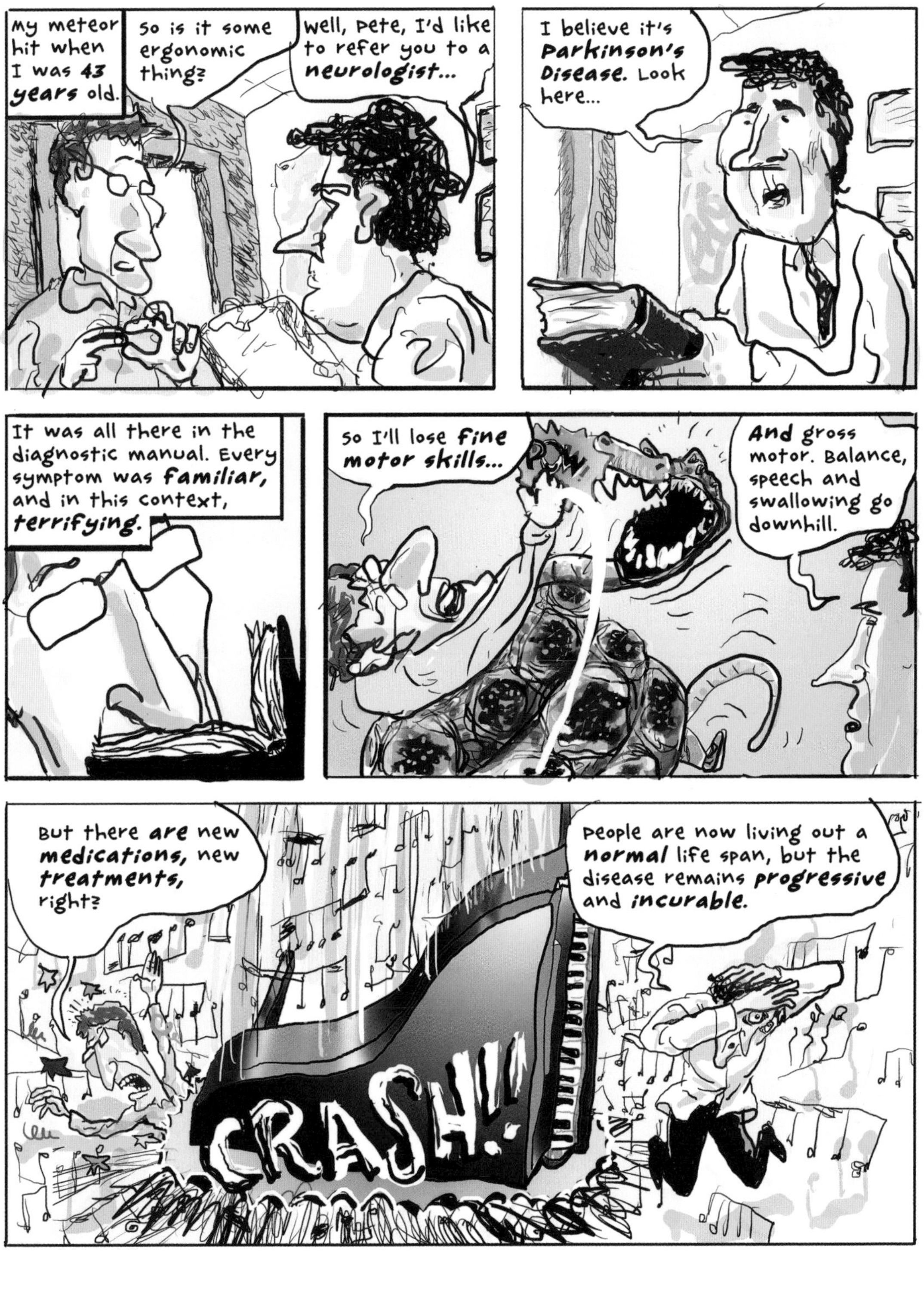
My meteor hit when I was 43 years old.
So is it some ergonomic thing?
Well, Pete, I'd like to refer you to a neurologist...
I believe it's Parkinson's Disease. Look here...
It was all there in the diagnostic manual. Every symptom was familiar, and in this context, terrifying.
So I'll lose fine motor skills...
And gross motor. Balance, speech and swallowing go downhill.
But there are new medications, new treatments, right?
People are now living out a normal life span, but the disease remains progressive and incurable.
CRASH!!

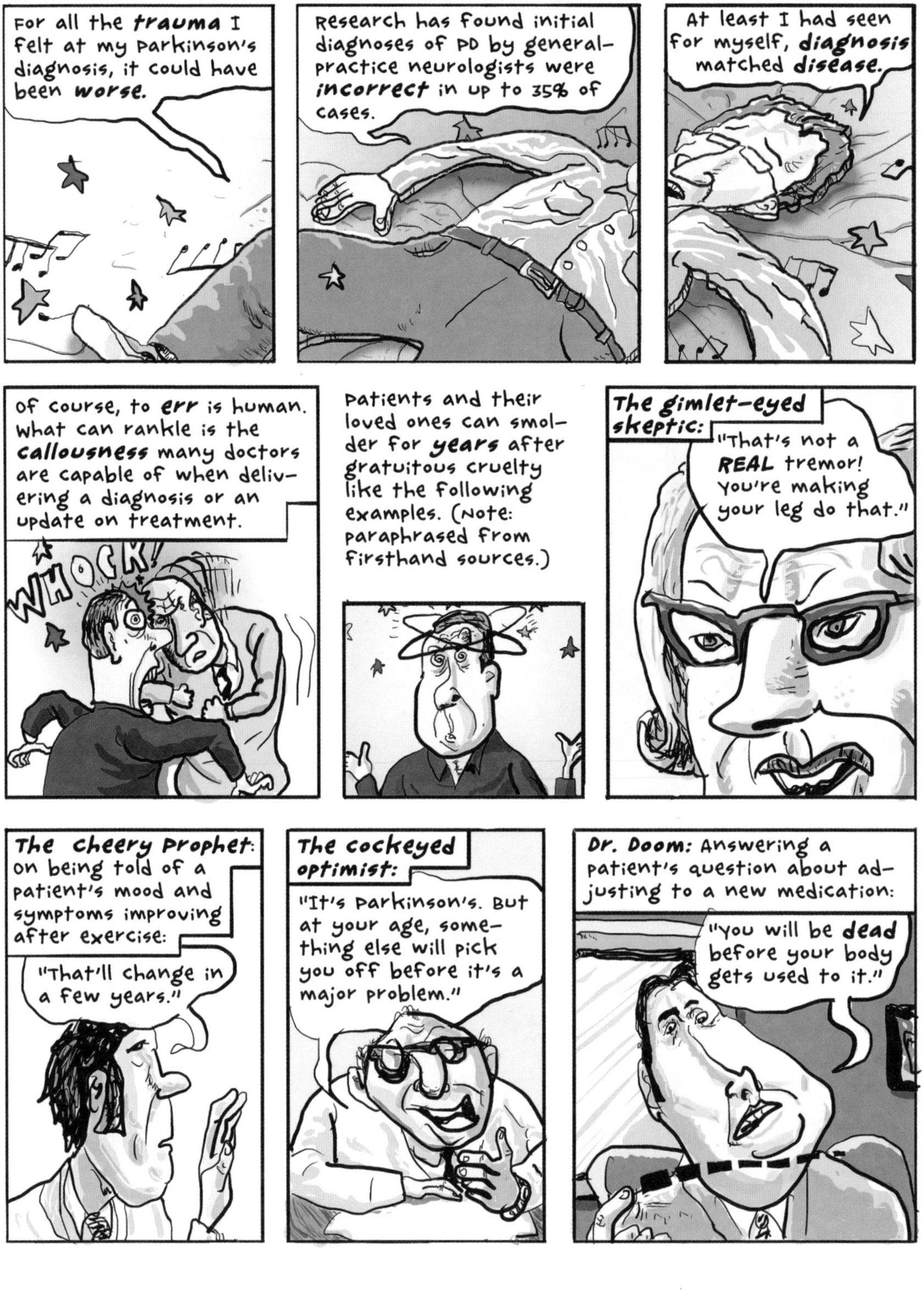
For all the *trauma* I felt at my Parkinson's diagnosis, it could have been *worse.*
Research has found initial diagnoses of PD by general-practice neurologists were *incorrect* in up to 35% of cases.
At least I had seen for myself, *diagnosis* matched *disease.*
Of course, to *err* is human. What can rankle is the *callousness* many doctors are capable of when delivering a diagnosis or an update on treatment.
WHOCK!
Patients and their loved ones can smolder for *years* after gratuitous cruelty like the following examples. (Note: paraphrased from firsthand sources.)
The gimlet-eyed skeptic:
"That's not a *REAL* tremor! You're making your leg do that."
The cheery prophet: on being told of a patient's mood and symptoms improving after exercise:
"That'll change in a few years."
The cockeyed optimist:
"It's Parkinson's. But at your age, something else will pick you off before it's a major problem."
Dr. Doom: Answering a patient's question about adjusting to a new medication:
"You will be *dead* before your body gets used to it."

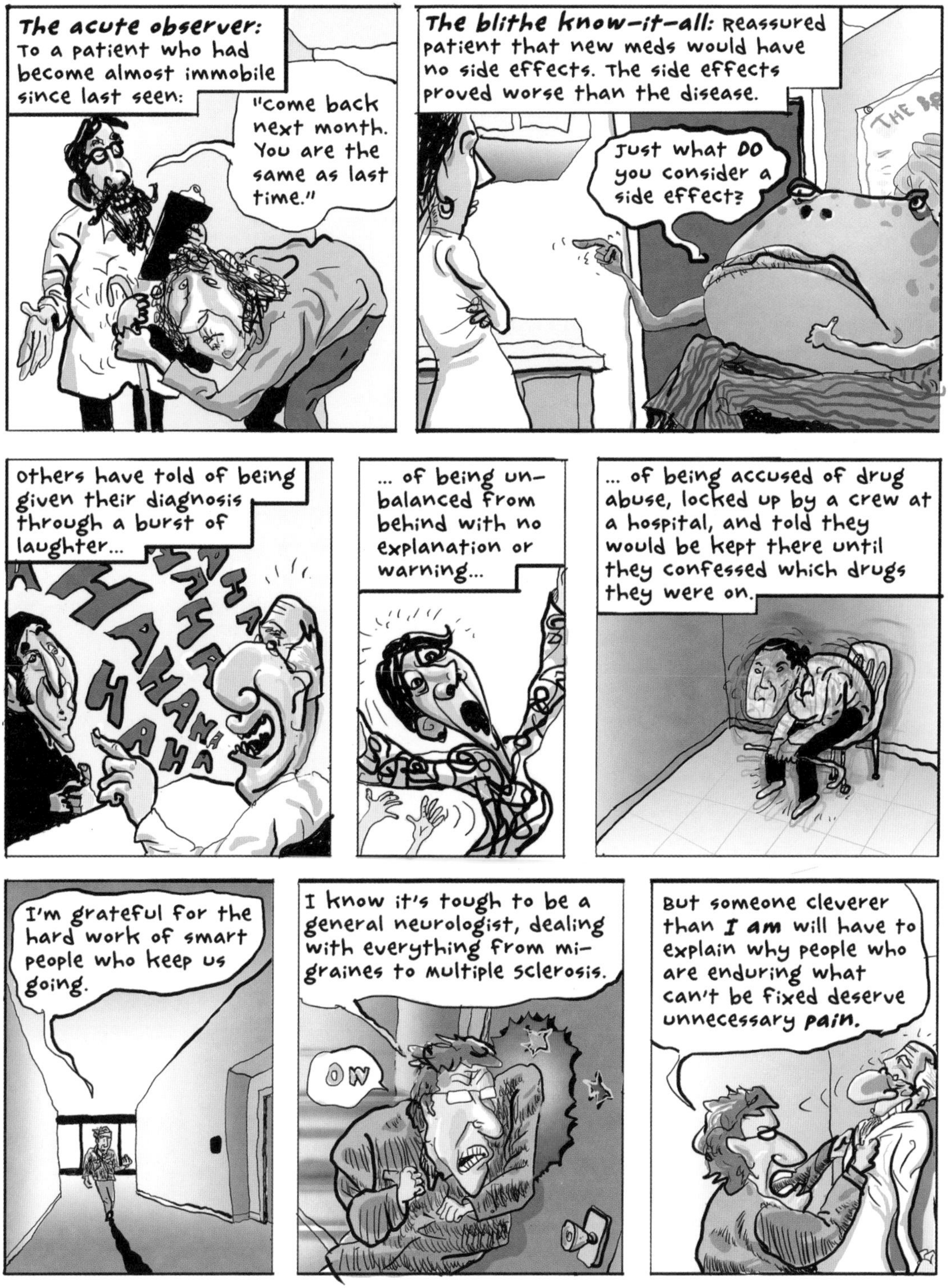
The acute observer: To a patient who had become almost immobile since last seen:
"Come back next month. You are the same as last time."
The blithe know-it-all: Reassured patient that new meds would have no side effects. The side effects proved worse than the disease.
Just what DO you consider a side effect?
Others have told of being given their diagnosis through a burst of laughter...
HAHAHAHAHAHA
... of being unbalanced from behind with no explanation or warning...
... of being accused of drug abuse, locked up by a crew at a hospital, and told they would be kept there until they confessed which drugs they were on.
I'm grateful for the hard work of smart people who keep us going.
I know it's tough to be a general neurologist, dealing with everything from migraines to multiple sclerosis.
OW
But someone cleverer than I am will have to explain why people who are enduring what can't be fixed deserve unnecessary pain.

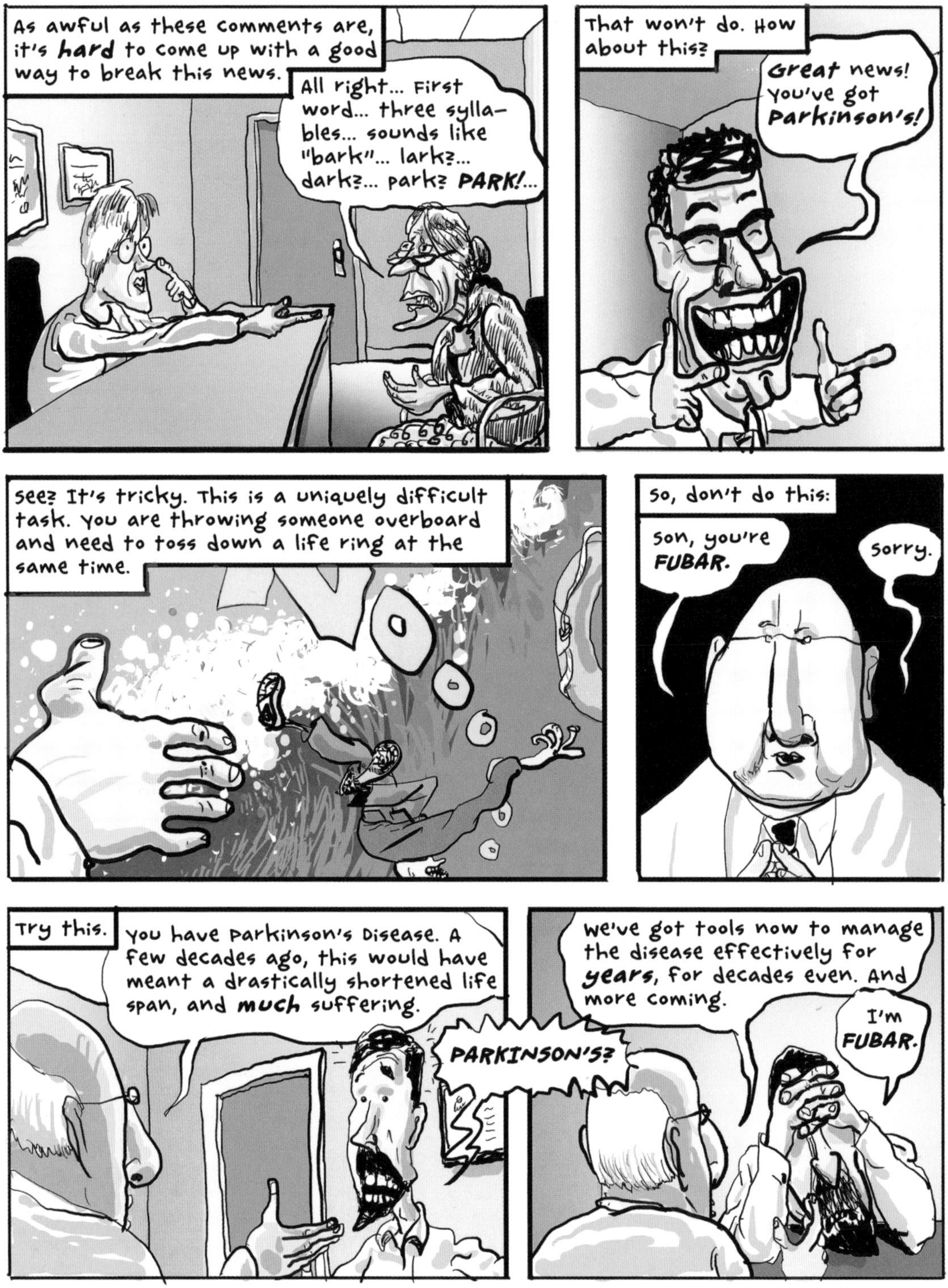

As awful as these comments are, it's **hard** to come up with a good way to break this news.
All right... First word... three sylla-bles... sounds like "bark"... lark?... dark?... park? **PARK!**...
That won't do. How about this?
Great news! You've got **Parkinson's!**
See? It's tricky. This is a uniquely difficult task. You are throwing someone overboard and need to toss down a life ring at the same time.
So, don't do this:
Son, you're **FUBAR**.
Sorry.
Try this.
You have Parkinson's Disease. A few decades ago, this would have meant a drastically shortened life span, and **much** suffering.
PARKINSON'S?
We've got tools now to manage the disease effectively for **years**, for decades even. And more coming.
I'm **FUBAR**.

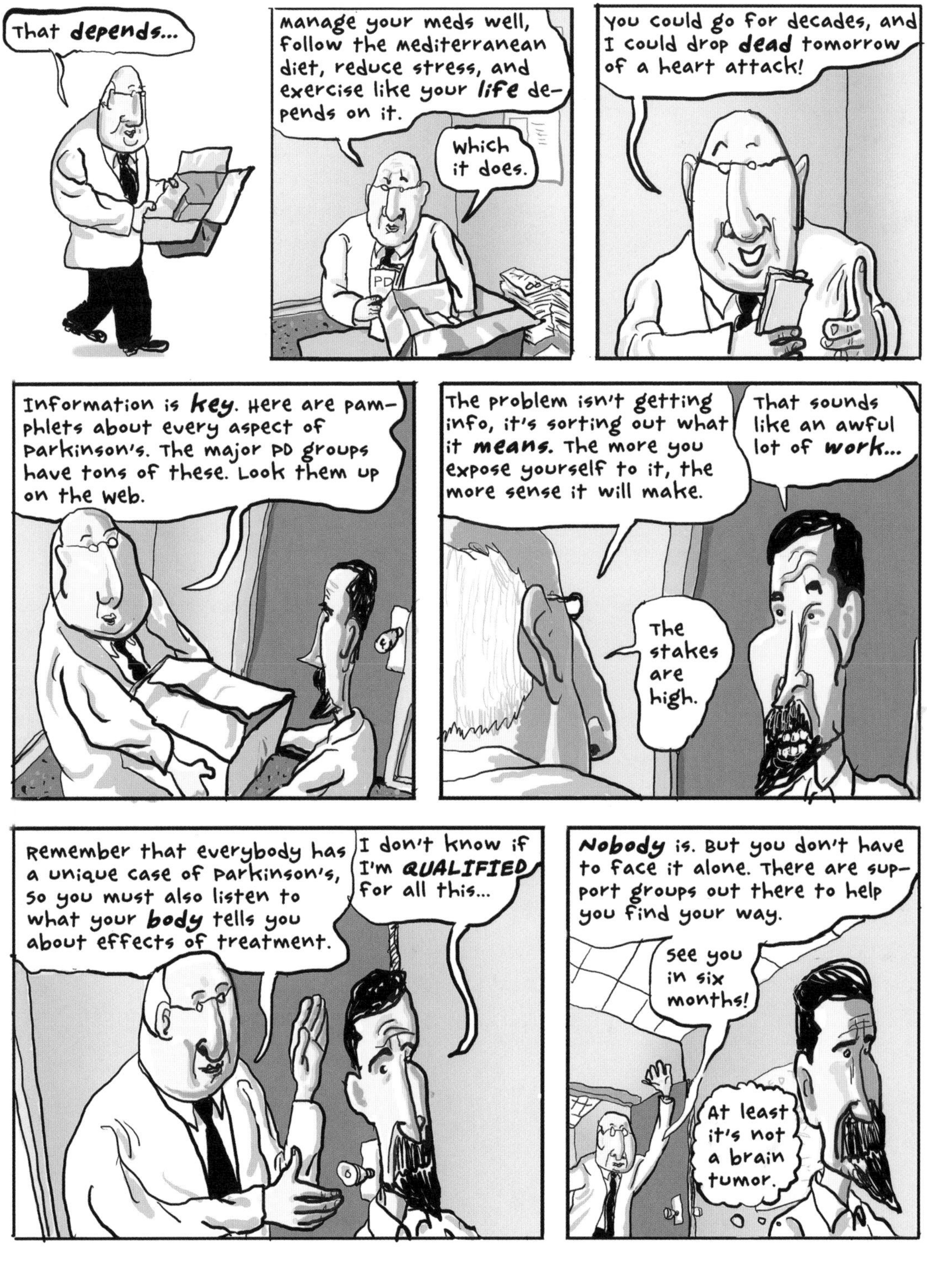

That **depends...**
manage your meds well, follow the mediterranean diet, reduce stress, and exercise like your ***life*** depends on it.
Which it does.
PD
You could go for decades, and I could drop **dead** tomorrow of a heart attack!
Information is ***key***. Here are pamphlets about every aspect of Parkinson's. The major PD groups have tons of these. Look them up on the web.
The problem isn't getting info, it's sorting out what it ***means***. The more you expose yourself to it, the more sense it will make.
That sounds like an awful lot of ***work...***
The stakes are high.
Remember that everybody has a unique case of Parkinson's, so you must also listen to what your ***body*** tells you about effects of treatment.
I don't know if I'm ***QUALIFIED*** for all this...
Nobody is. But you don't have to face it alone. There are support groups out there to help you find your way.
See you in six months!
At least it's not a brain tumor.

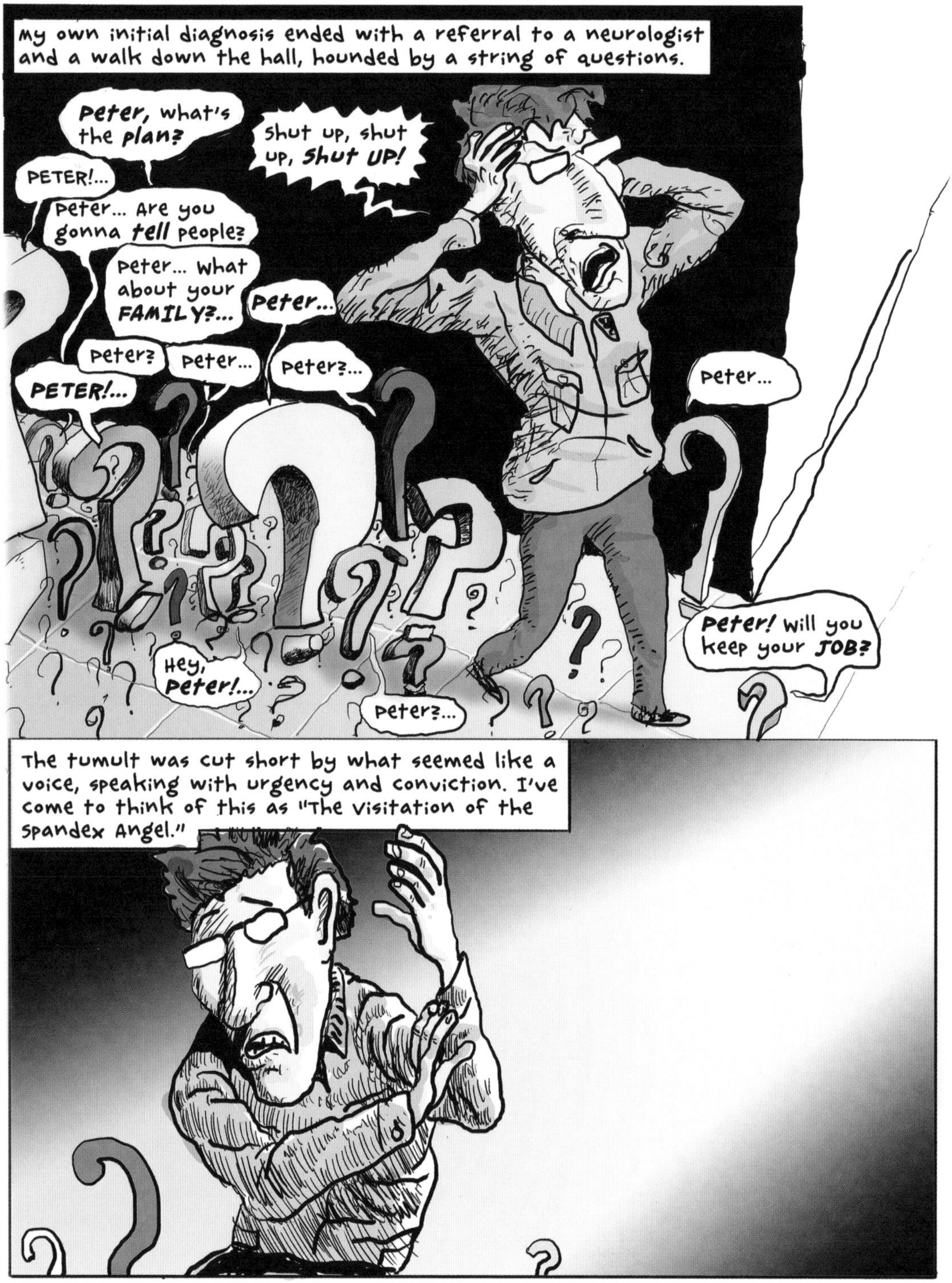
My own initial diagnosis ended with a referral to a neurologist and a walk down the hall, hounded by a string of questions.
Peter, what's the plan?
Shut up, shut up, Shut UP!
PETER!...
Peter... Are you gonna tell people?
Peter... What about your FAMILY?...
Peter...
Peter?
Peter...
Peter?...
PETER!...
Peter...
Hey, Peter!...
Peter?...
Peter! Will you keep your JOB?
The tumult was cut short by what seemed like a voice, speaking with urgency and conviction. I've come to think of this as "The Visitation of the Spandex Angel."

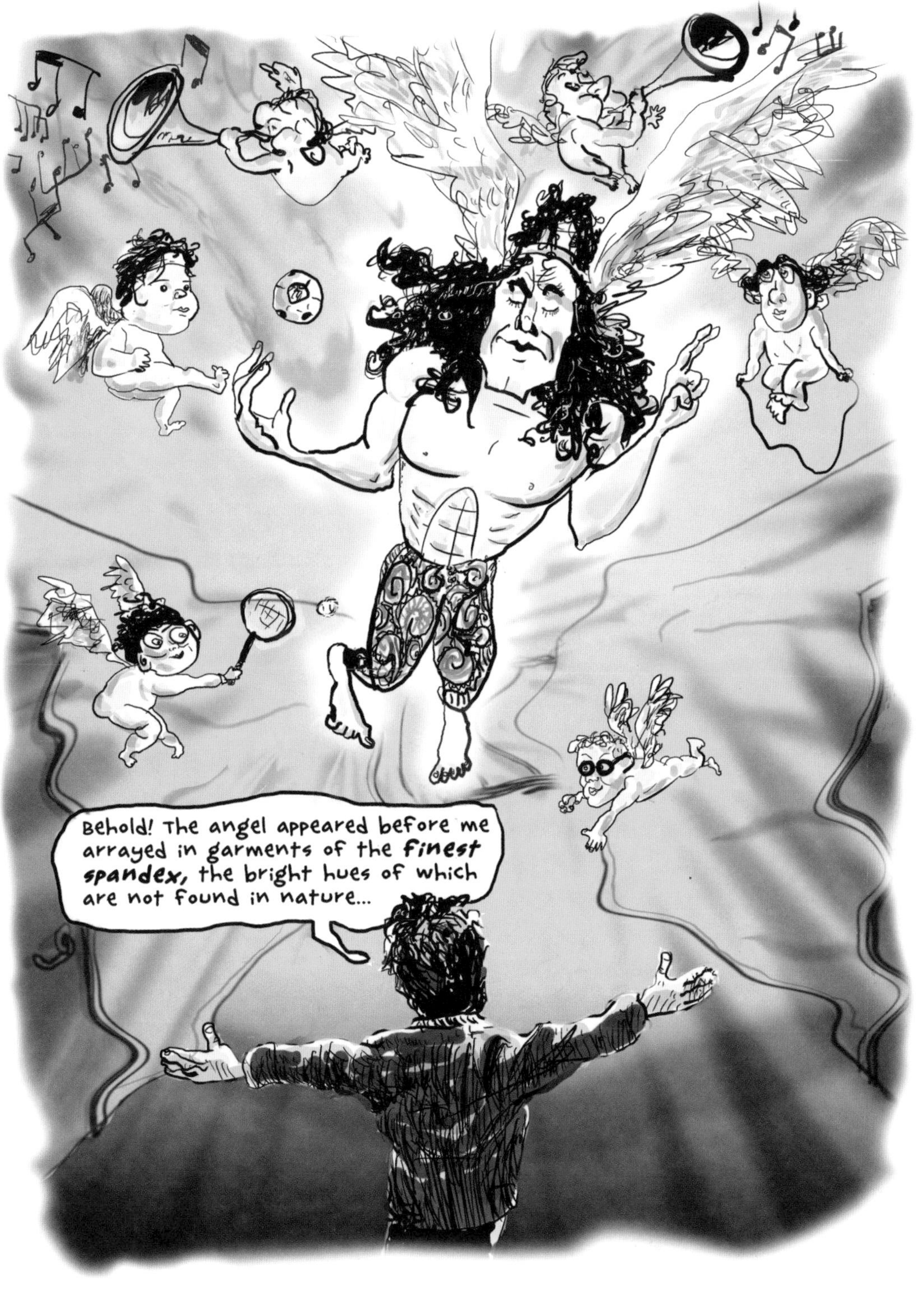
Behold! The angel appeared before me arrayed in garments of the finest spandex, the bright hues of which are not found in nature...

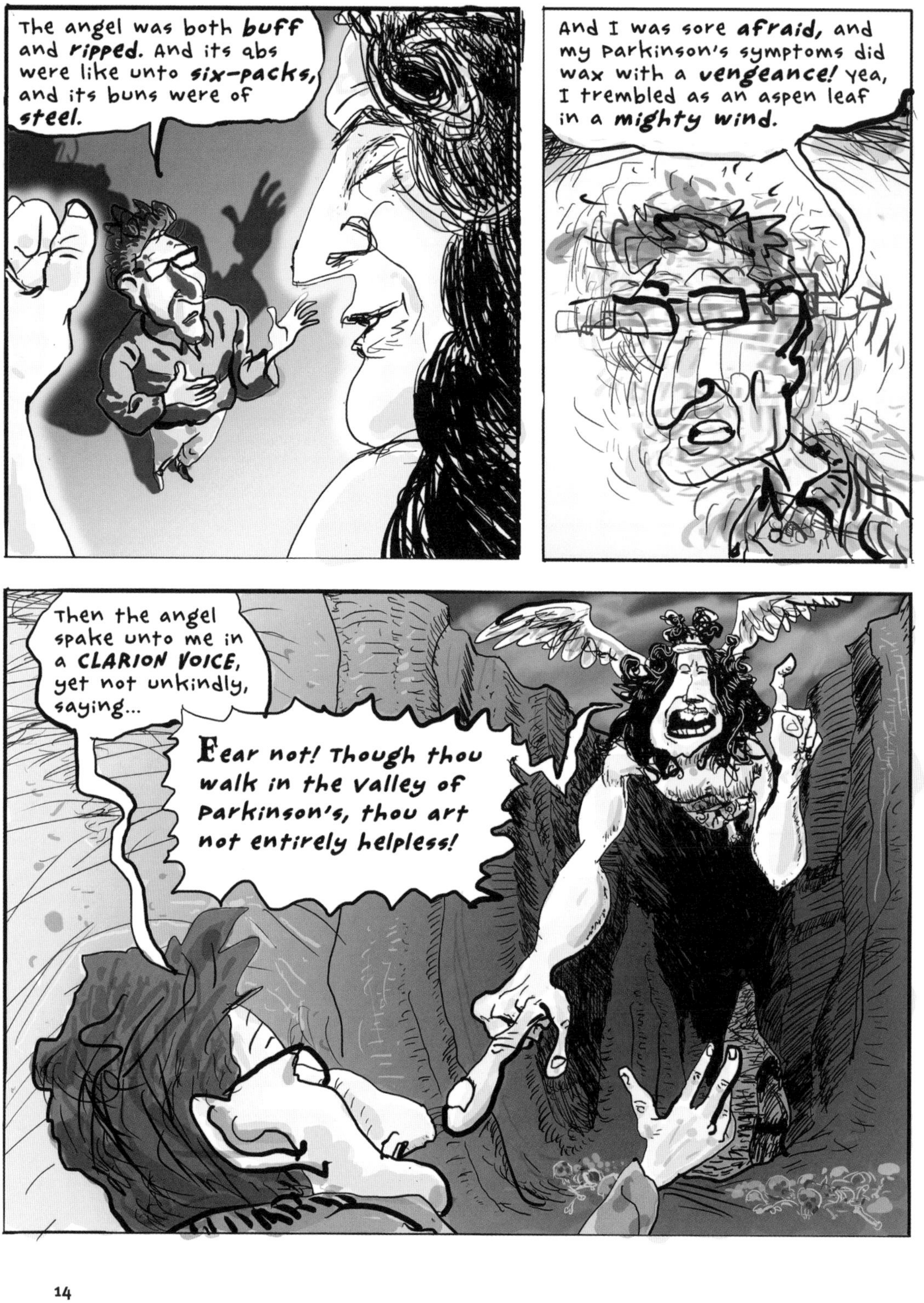
The angel was both buff and ripped. And its abs were like unto six-packs, and its buns were of steel.
And I was sore afraid, and my Parkinson's symptoms did wax with a vengeance! Yea, I trembled as an aspen leaf in a mighty wind.
Then the angel spake unto me in a CLARION VOICE, yet not unkindly, saying...
Fear not! Though thou walk in the valley of Parkinson's, thou art not entirely helpless!

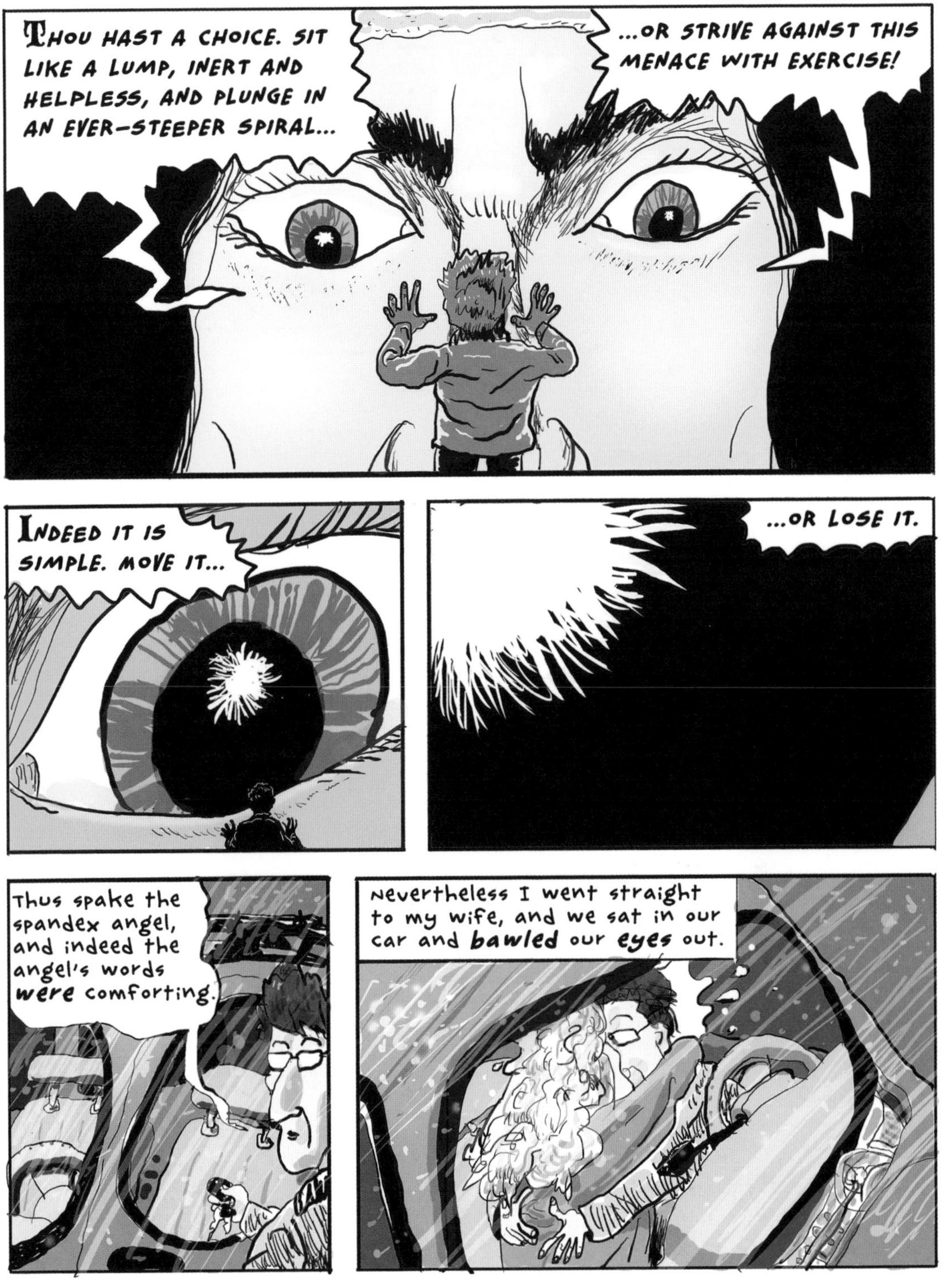
Thou hast a choice. Sit like a lump, inert and helpless, and plunge in an ever-steeper spiral...
...or strive against this menace with exercise!
Indeed it is simple. Move it...
...or lose it.
Thus spake the spandex angel, and indeed the angel's words were comforting.
Nevertheless I went straight to my wife, and we sat in our car and bawled our eyes out.

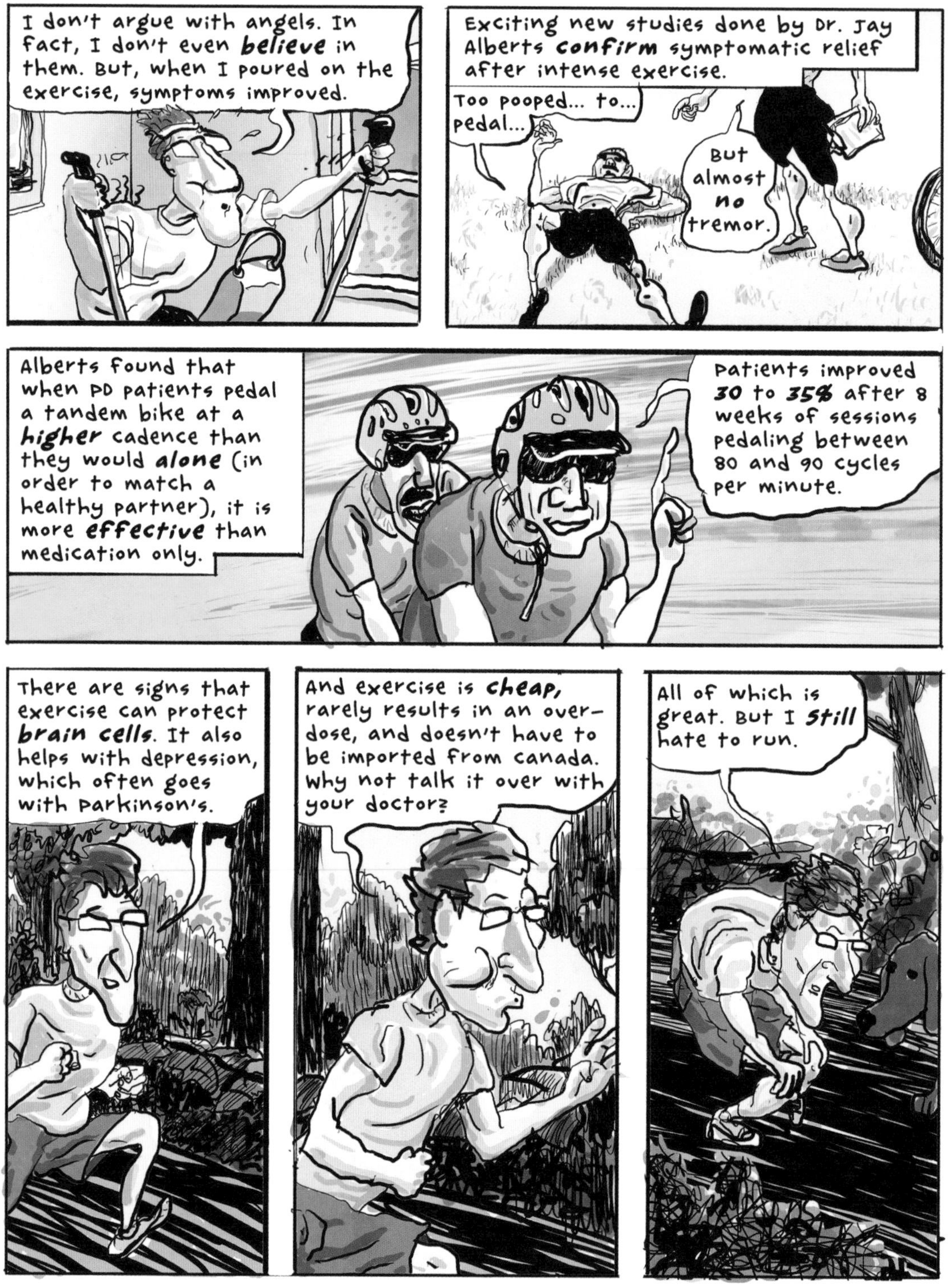
I don't argue with angels. In fact, I don't even believe in them. But, when I poured on the exercise, symptoms improved.
Exciting new studies done by Dr. Jay Alberts confirm symptomatic relief after intense exercise.
Too pooped... to... pedal...
But almost no tremor.
Alberts found that when PD patients pedal a tandem bike at a higher cadence than they would alone (in order to match a healthy partner), it is more effective than medication only.
Patients improved 30 to 35% after 8 weeks of sessions pedaling between 80 and 90 cycles per minute.
There are signs that exercise can protect brain cells. It also helps with depression, which often goes with Parkinson's.
And exercise is cheap, rarely results in an over-dose, and doesn't have to be imported from Canada. Why not talk it over with your doctor?
All of which is great. But I still hate to run.

2. Learning to Speak Parkinson's

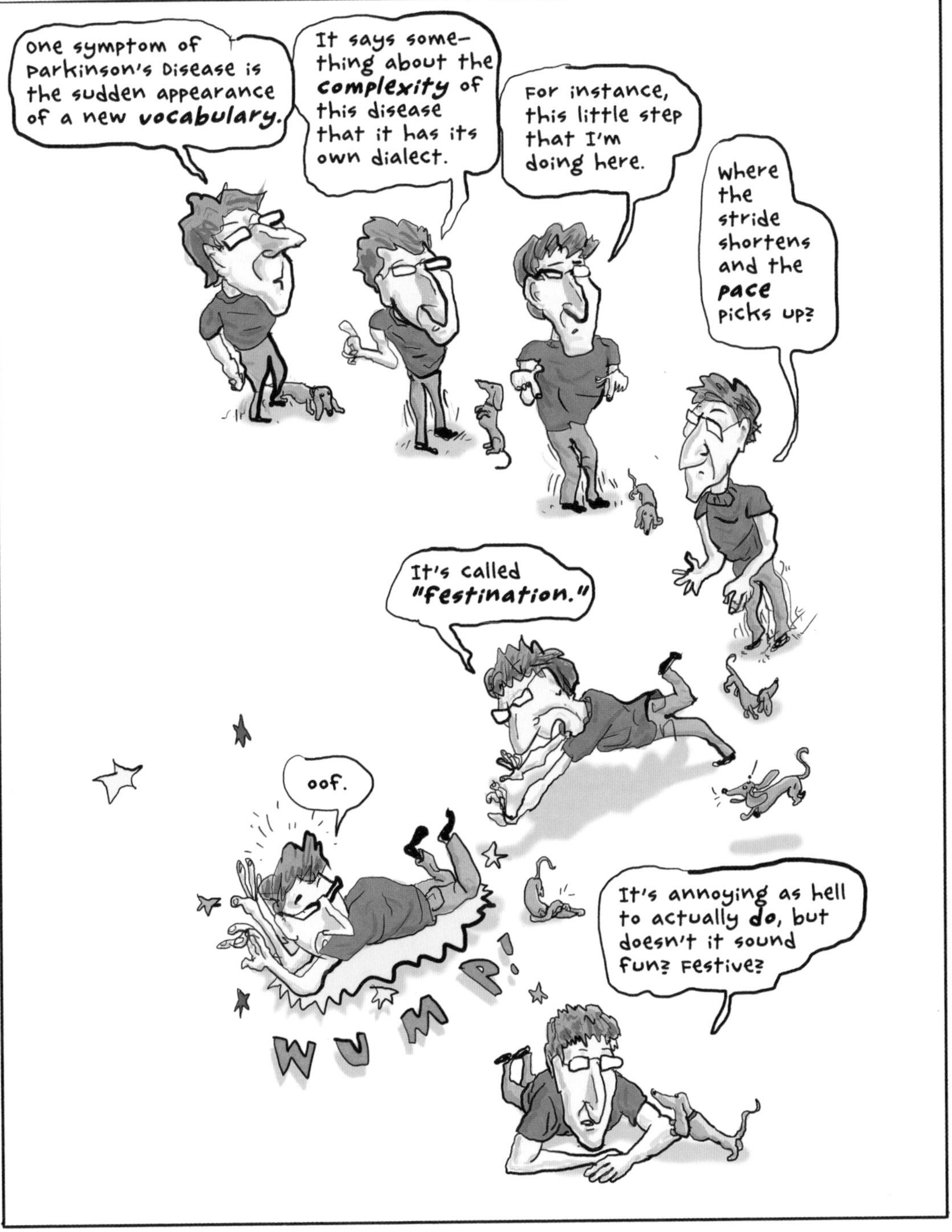
One symptom of Parkinson's Disease is the sudden appearance of a new vocabulary.
It says some-thing about the complexity of this disease that it has its own dialect.
For instance, this little step that I'm doing here.
Where the stride shortens and the pace picks up?
It's called "festination."
oof.
WUMP!
It's annoying as hell to actually do, but doesn't it sound fun? Festive?

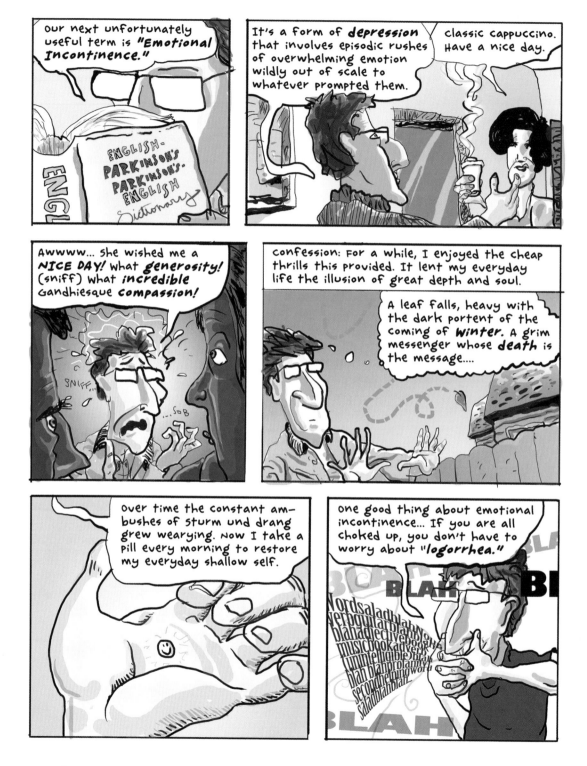

Our next unfortunately useful term is "Emotional Incontinence."

ENGLISH-PARKINSON'S-PARKINSON'S-ENGLISH Dictionary

It's a form of **depression** that involves episodic rushes of overwhelming emotion wildly out of scale to whatever prompted them.

Classic cappuccino. Have a nice day.

Awwww... she wished me a **NICE DAY!** What **generosity!** (sniff) What **incredible** Gandhiesque **compassion!**

SNIFF...

...SOB

Confession: For a while, I enjoyed the cheap thrills this provided. It lent my everyday life the illusion of great depth and soul.

A leaf falls, heavy with the dark portent of the coming of **winter**. A grim messenger whose **death** is the message....

Over time the constant ambushes of sturm und drang grew wearying. Now I take a pill every morning to restore my everyday shallow self.

One good thing about emotional incontinence... If you are all choked up, you don't have to worry about "logorrhea."

BLAH wordsalad blah verbgular blah noun blah adjective boohoo musicbook ad year unintelligible blah blah profamily second helping word salad blah blah blah BLAH

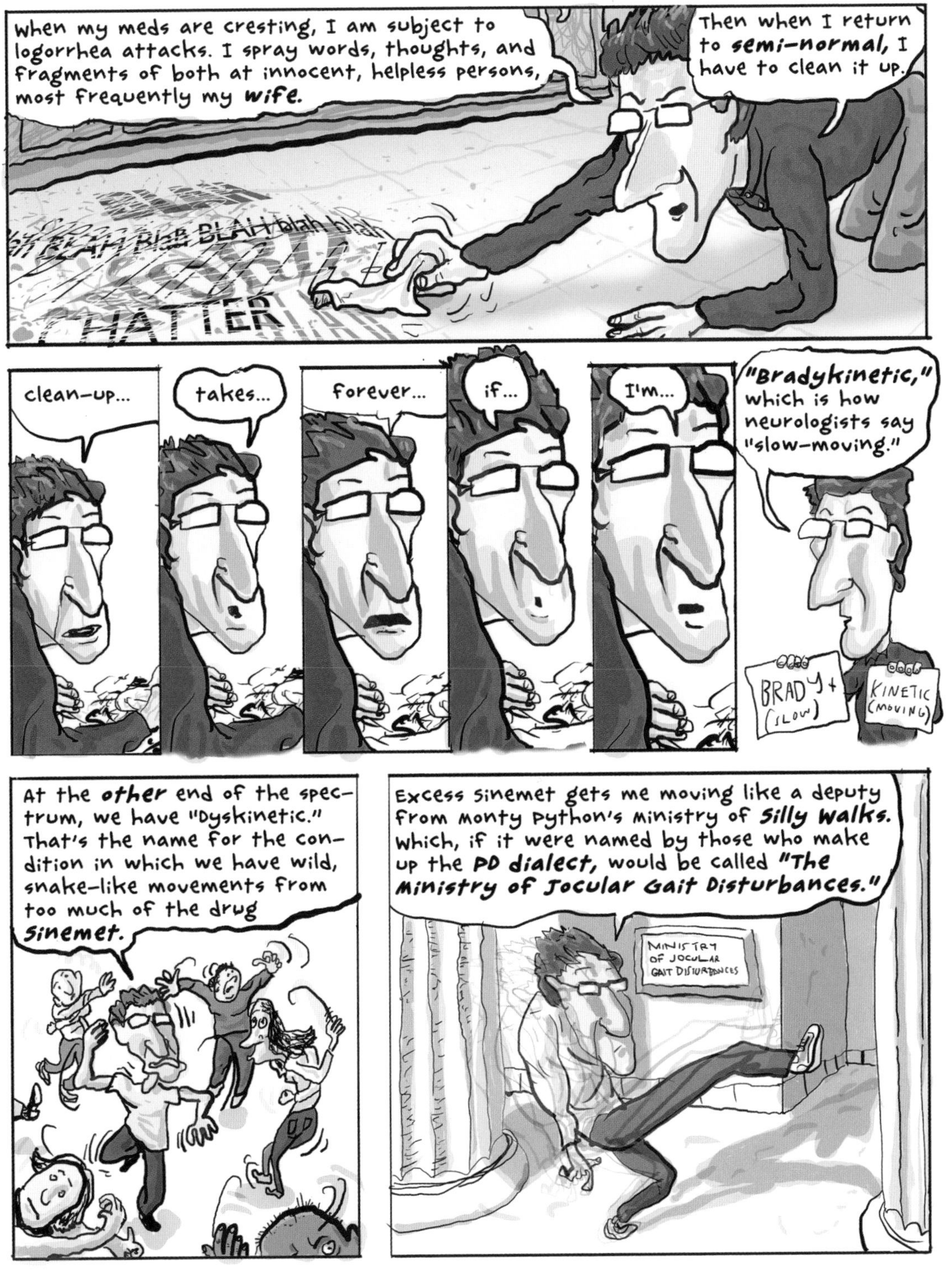
When my meds are cresting, I am subject to logorrhea attacks. I spray words, thoughts, and fragments of both at innocent, helpless persons, most frequently my **wife.**
Then when I return to **semi-normal,** I have to clean it up.
BLAH Blah BLAH blah blah
CHATTER
clean-up...
takes...
forever...
if...
I'm...
"Bradykinetic," which is how neurologists say "slow-moving."
BRADY + (SLOW)
KINETIC (MOVING)
At the **other** end of the spectrum, we have "Dyskinetic." That's the name for the condition in which we have wild, snake-like movements from too much of the drug **sinemet.**
Excess sinemet gets me moving like a deputy from Monty Python's Ministry of **Silly Walks.** Which, if it were named by those who make up the **PD dialect,** would be called **"The Ministry of Jocular Gait Disturbances."**
MINISTRY OF JOCULAR GAIT DISTURBANCES

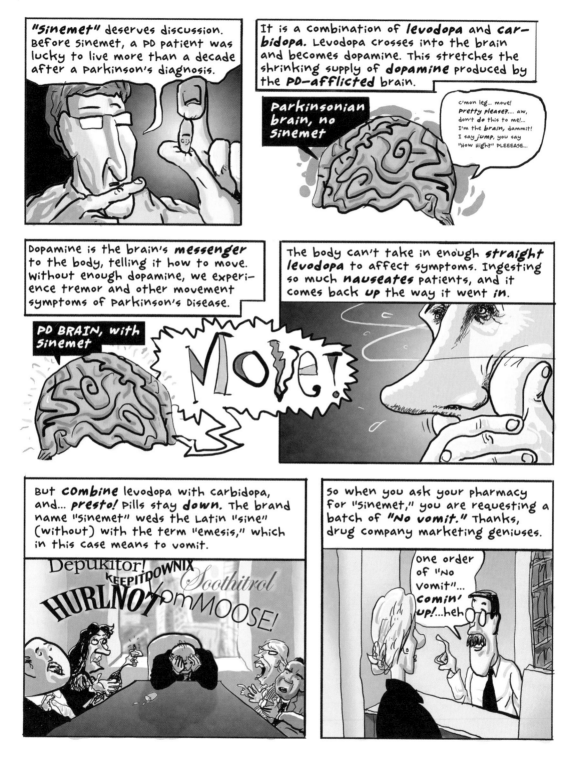

"Sinemet" deserves discussion. Before sinemet, a PD patient was lucky to live more than a decade after a Parkinson's diagnosis.

It is a combination of **levodopa** and **carbidopa**. Levodopa crosses into the brain and becomes dopamine. This stretches the shrinking supply of **dopamine** produced by the **PD-afflicted** brain.

Parkinsonian brain, no sinemet

c'mon leg... move! *Pretty please?*... aw, don't *do* this to me!... I'm the *brain*, dammit! I say *jump*, you say "How *High*?" PLEEEASE...

Dopamine is the brain's **messenger** to the body, telling it how to move. Without enough dopamine, we experience tremor and other movement symptoms of Parkinson's Disease.

The body can't take in enough **straight levodopa** to affect symptoms. Ingesting so much **nauseates** patients, and it comes back **up** the way it went **in**.

PD BRAIN, with sinemet

MOVE!

But **combine** levodopa with carbidopa, and... **presto!** Pills stay **down**. The brand name "sinemet" weds the Latin "sine" (without) with the term "emesis," which in this case means to vomit.

Depukitor! KEEPITDOWNIX Soothitrol HURLNOT VomMOOSE!

So when you ask your pharmacy for "sinemet," you are requesting a batch of **"No vomit."** Thanks, drug company marketing geniuses.

One order of "No Vomit"... **comin' up!**...heh

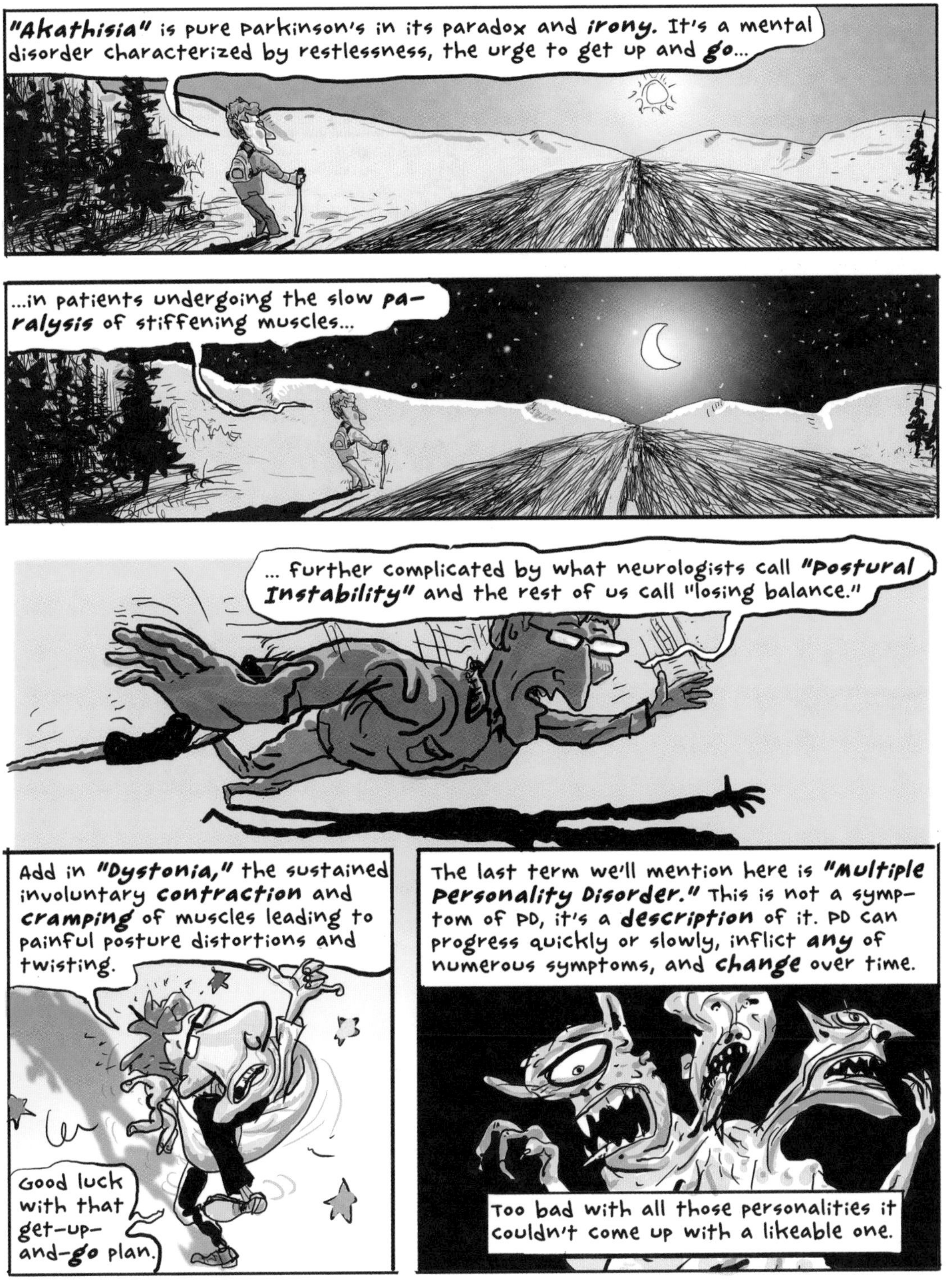
"Akathisia" is pure Parkinson's in its paradox and irony. It's a mental disorder characterized by restlessness, the urge to get up and go...
...in patients undergoing the slow paralysis of stiffening muscles...
... further complicated by what neurologists call "Postural Instability" and the rest of us call "losing balance."
Add in "Dystonia," the sustained involuntary contraction and cramping of muscles leading to painful posture distortions and twisting.
Good luck with that get-up-and-go plan.
The last term we'll mention here is "Multiple Personality Disorder." This is not a symptom of PD, it's a description of it. PD can progress quickly or slowly, inflict any of numerous symptoms, and change over time.
Too bad with all those personalities it couldn't come up with a likeable one.

3. Interview with a Killer

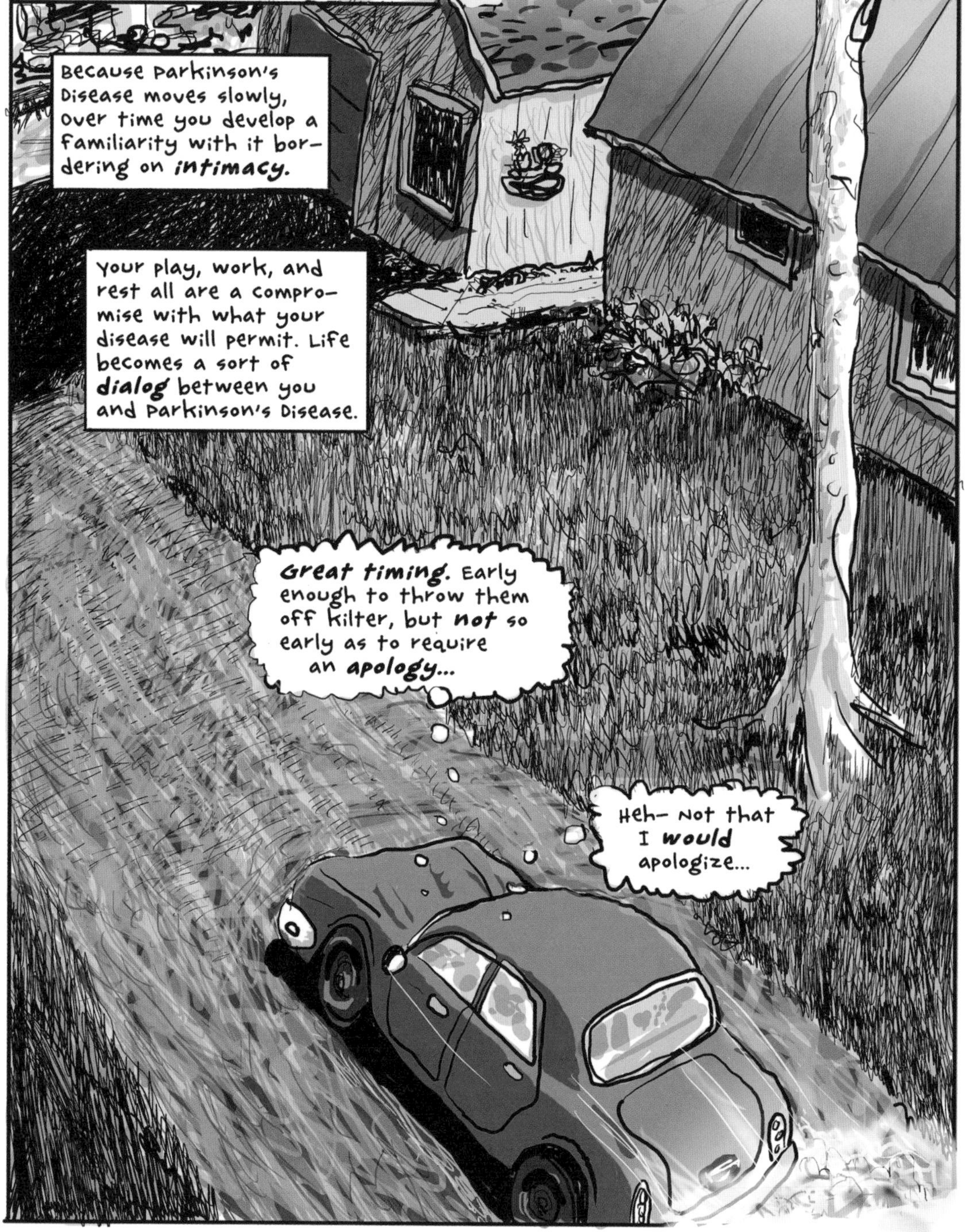
Because Parkinson's Disease moves slowly, over time you develop a familiarity with it bordering on *intimacy.*
Your play, work, and rest all are a compromise with what your disease will permit. Life becomes a sort of ***dialog*** between you and Parkinson's Disease.
Great timing. Early enough to throw them off kilter, but ***not*** so early as to require an ***apology...***
Heh– Not that I ***would*** apologize...

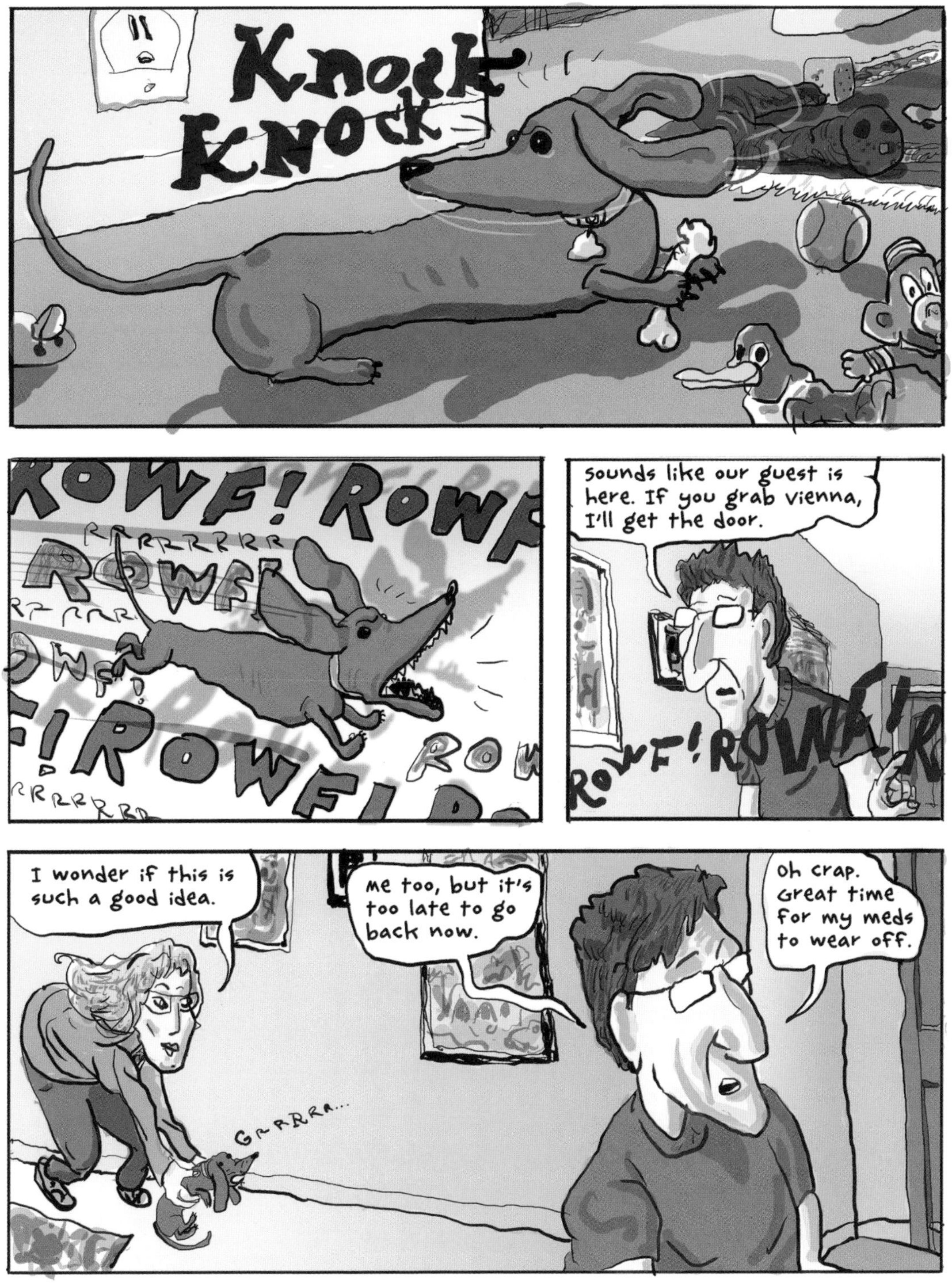
Knock
Knock
ROWF! ROWF
RRRRRRRRR
ROWF!
ROWF!
ROW
sounds like our guest is here. If you grab vienna, I'll get the door.
ROWF! ROWF! R
I wonder if this is such a good idea.
me too, but it's too late to go back now.
oh crap. Great time for my meds to wear off.
GRRRRR...

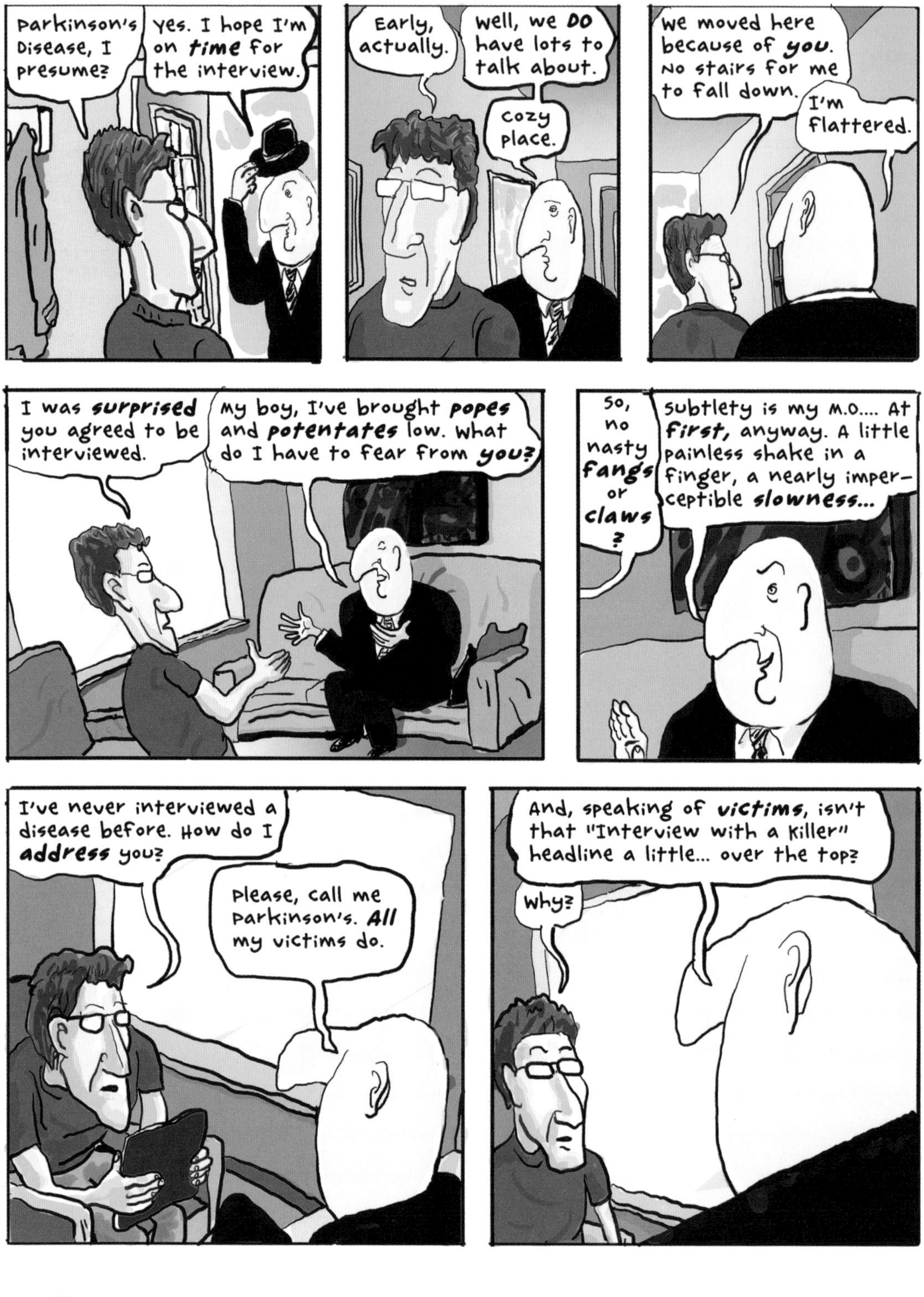
Parkinson's Disease, I presume?
Yes. I hope I'm on time for the interview.
Early, actually.
Well, we DO have lots to talk about.
Cozy place.
We moved here because of you. No stairs for me to fall down.
I'm flattered.
I was surprised you agreed to be interviewed.
My boy, I've brought popes and potentates low. What do I have to fear from you?
So, no nasty fangs or claws?
Subtlety is my M.O.... At first, anyway. A little painless shake in a finger, a nearly imperceptible slowness...
I've never interviewed a disease before. How do I address you?
Please, call me Parkinson's. All my victims do.
And, speaking of victims, isn't that "Interview with a Killer" headline a little... over the top?
Why?

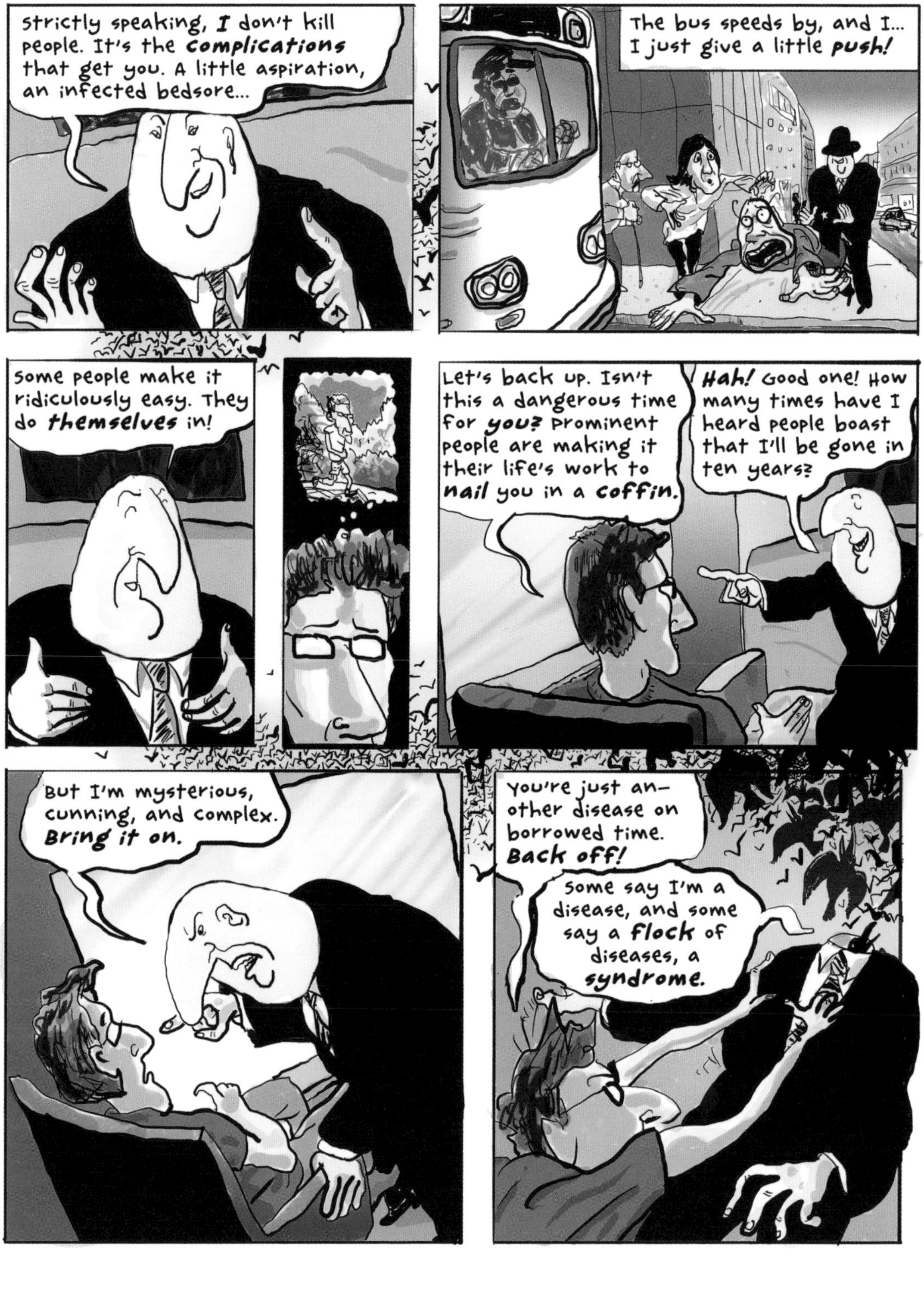
Strictly speaking, I don't kill people. It's the complications that get you. A little aspiration, an infected bedsore...
The bus speeds by, and I... I just give a little push!
Some people make it ridiculously easy. They do themselves in!
Let's back up. Isn't this a dangerous time for you? Prominent people are making it their life's work to nail you in a coffin.
Hah! Good one! How many times have I heard people boast that I'll be gone in ten years?
But I'm mysterious, cunning, and complex. Bring it on.
You're just another disease on borrowed time. Back off!
Some say I'm a disease, and some say a flock of diseases, a syndrome.

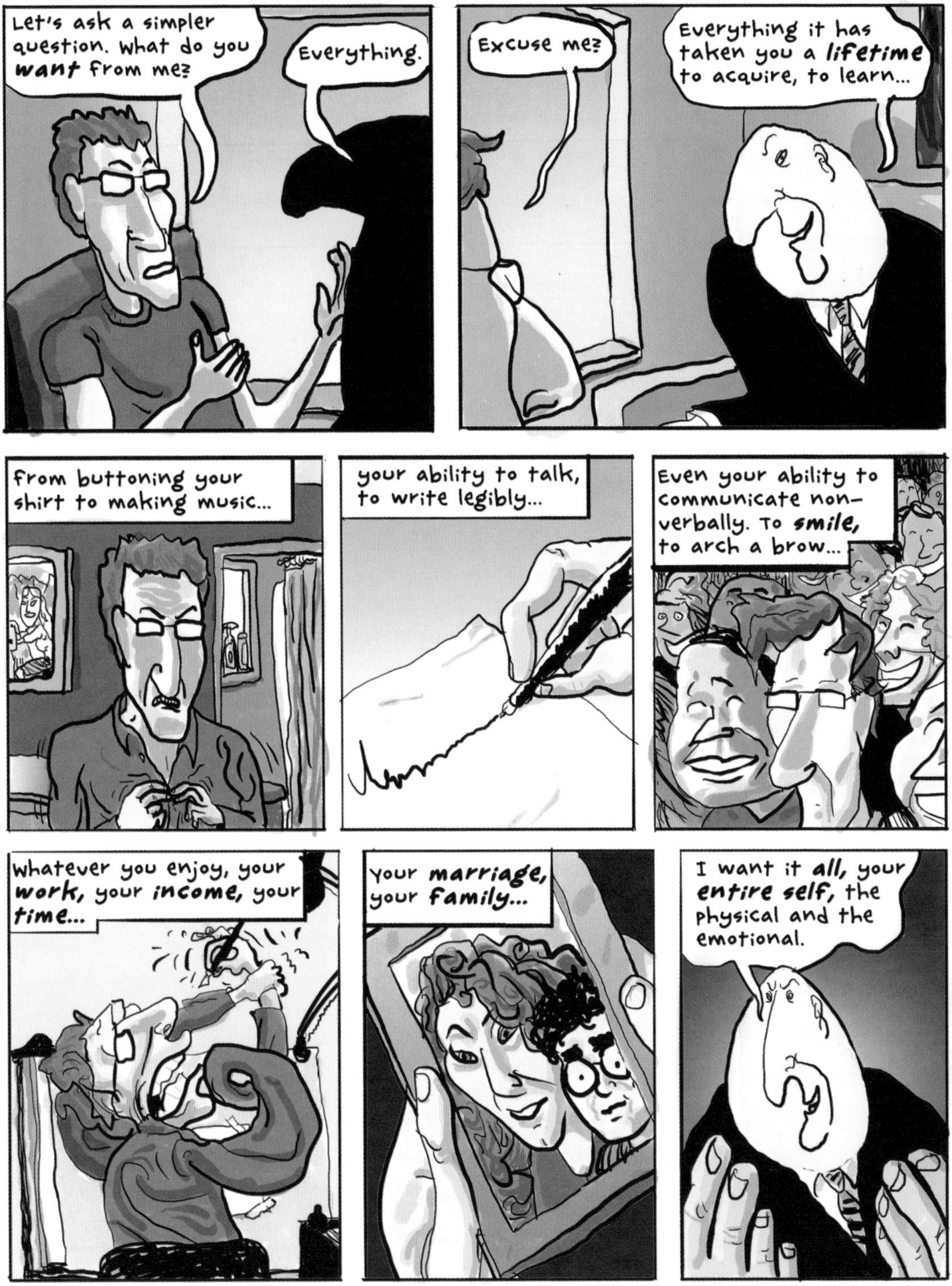
Let's ask a simpler question. What do you want from me?
Everything.
Excuse me?
Everything it has taken you a lifetime to acquire, to learn...
From buttoning your shirt to making music...
your ability to talk, to write legibly...
Even your ability to communicate non-verbally. To smile, to arch a brow...
whatever you enjoy, your work, your income, your time...
Your marriage, your family...
I want it all, your entire self, the physical and the emotional.

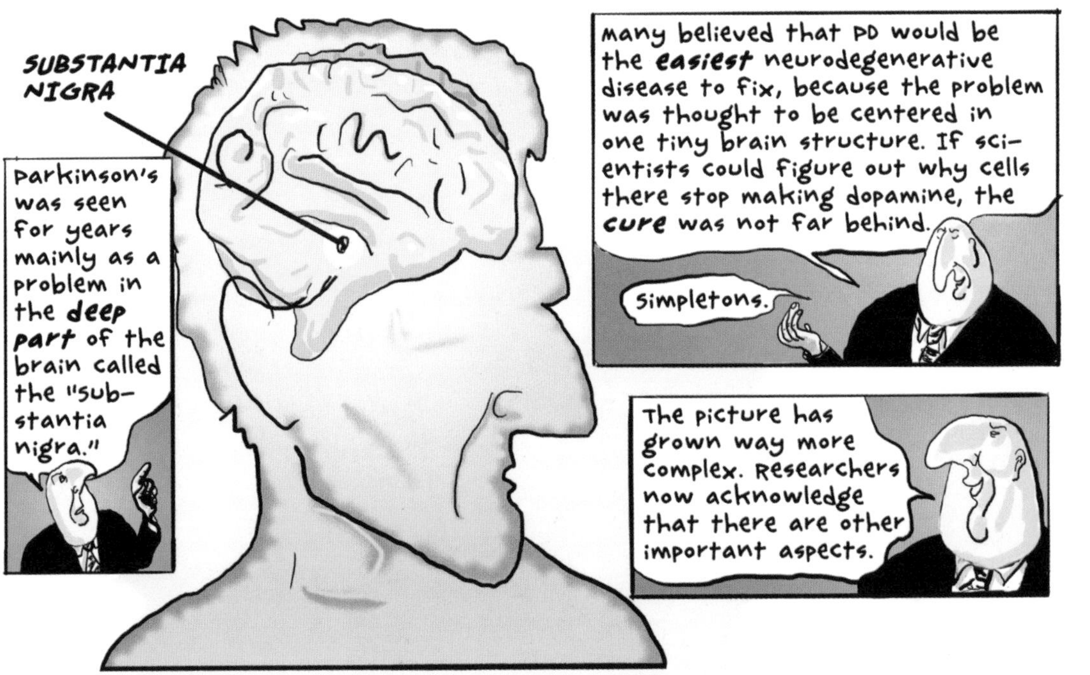
SUBSTANTIA NIGRA
Parkinson's was seen for years mainly as a problem in the deep part of the brain called the "substantia nigra."
many believed that PD would be the easiest neurodegenerative disease to fix, because the problem was thought to be centered in one tiny brain structure. If scientists could figure out why cells there stop making dopamine, the cure was not far behind.
Simpletons.
The picture has grown way more complex. Researchers now acknowledge that there are other important aspects.

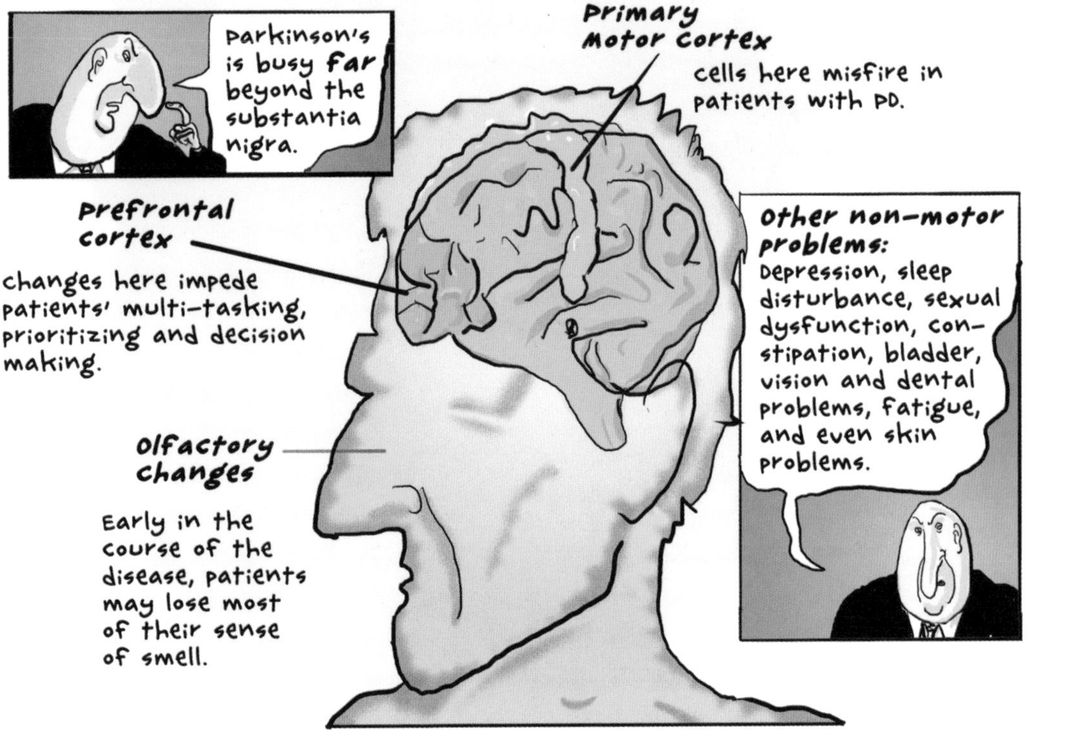
Parkinson's is busy far beyond the substantia nigra.
Primary motor cortex
cells here misfire in patients with PD.
Prefrontal cortex
changes here impede patients' multi-tasking, prioritizing and decision making.
Olfactory changes
Early in the course of the disease, patients may lose most of their sense of smell.
Other non-motor problems:
Depression, sleep disturbance, sexual dysfunction, constipation, bladder, vision and dental problems, fatigue, and even skin problems.

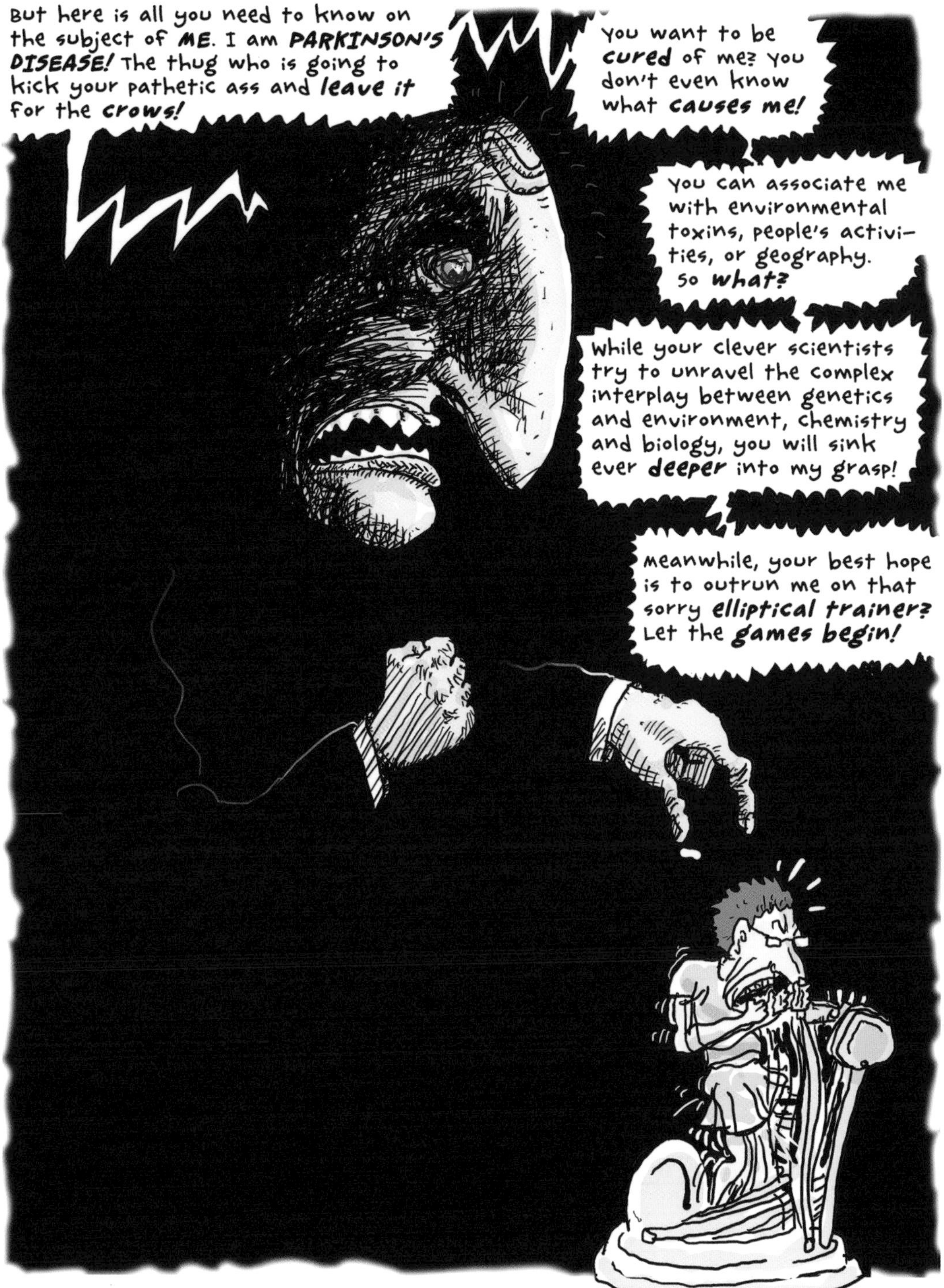
But here is all you need to know on the subject of ME. I am PARKINSON'S DISEASE! The thug who is going to kick your pathetic ass and leave it for the crows!
You want to be cured of me? You don't even know what causes me!
You can associate me with environmental toxins, people's activities, or geography. So what?
While your clever scientists try to unravel the complex interplay between genetics and environment, chemistry and biology, you will sink ever deeper into my grasp!
Meanwhile, your best hope is to outrun me on that sorry elliptical trainer? Let the games begin!

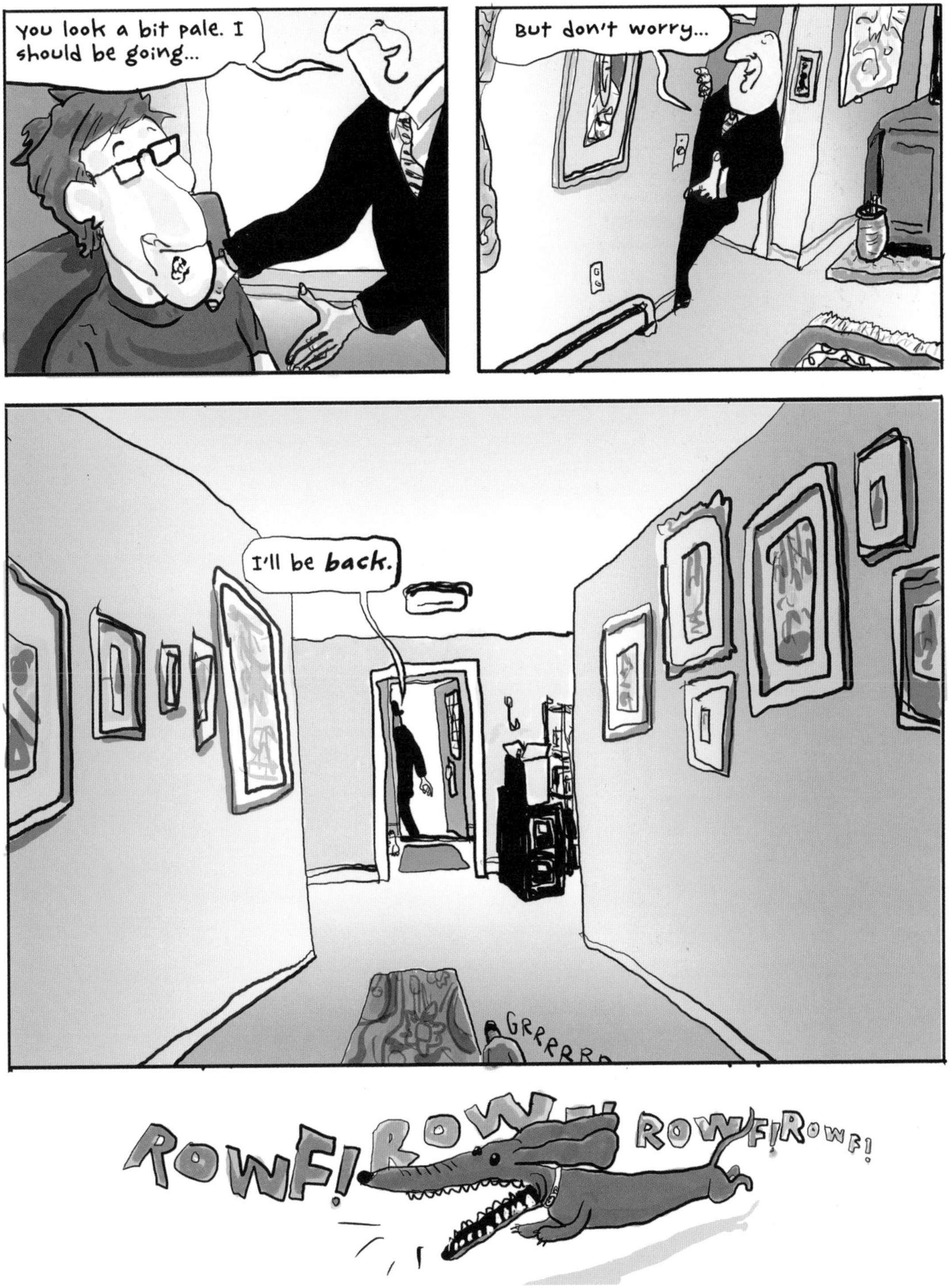
you look a bit pale. I should be going...
But don't worry...
I'll be **back.**
GRRRRRR
ROWF!
ROWF!ROWF!

4. Moping and Coping

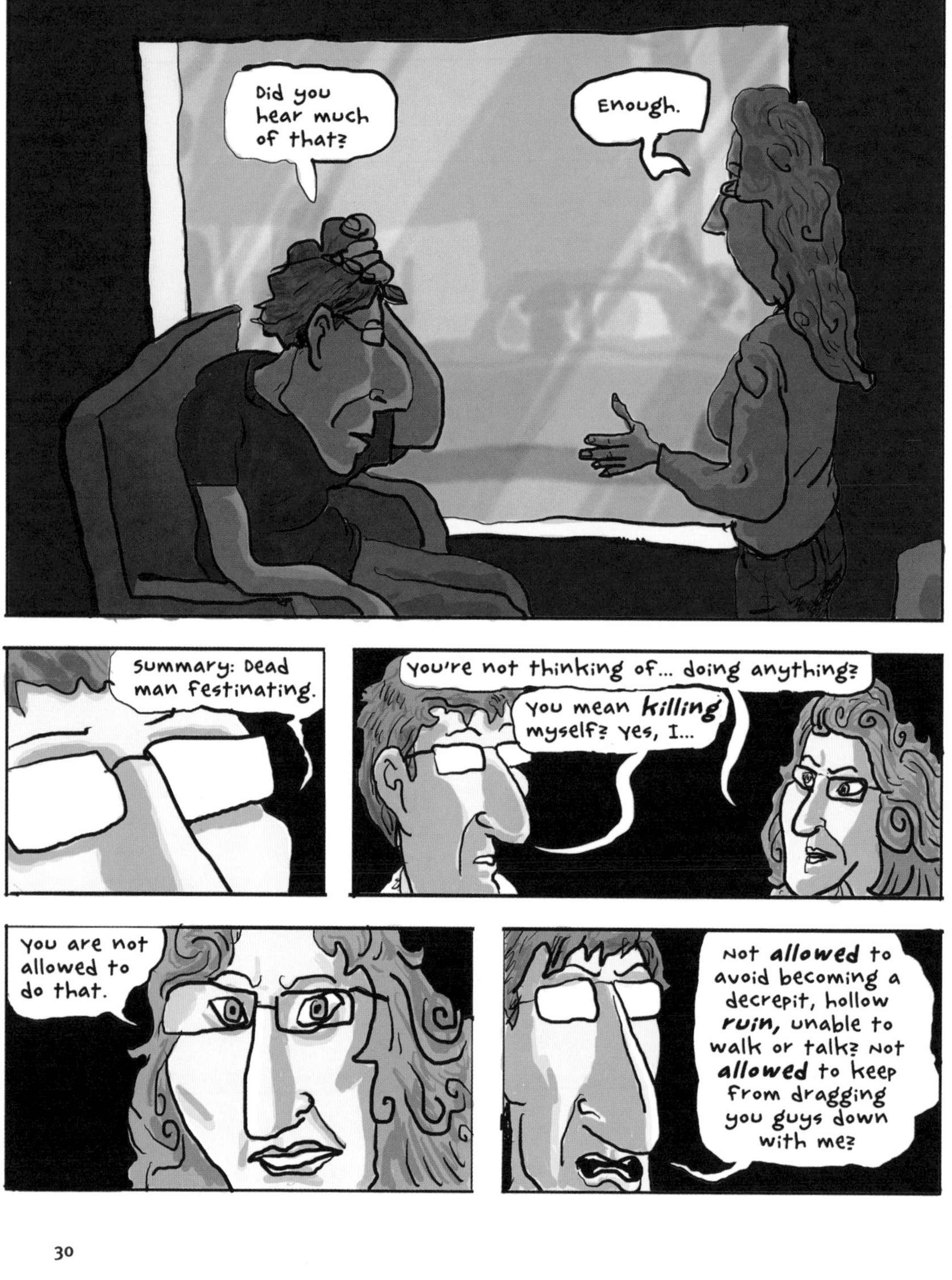
Did you hear much of that?
Enough.
Summary: Dead man festinating.
You're not thinking of... doing anything?
You mean **killing** myself? Yes, I...
You are not allowed to do that.
Not **allowed** to avoid becoming a decrepit, hollow **ruin,** unable to walk or talk? Not **allowed** to keep from dragging you guys down with me?

Not **allowed** to prevent wiley's memory of his father from being an image of a drooling ghost haunting the body that overthrew him?

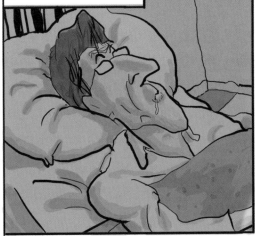

A cartoonist who couldn't **draw?** A guitar player who couldn't **play?** A **loser** who forced his family into **poverty** to house a shell that wasn't even him anymore in some **institutional home...**

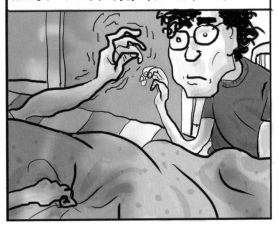

Diapered, mute, dependent on the whims and leisure of others to even get outside, feel the **sun** and **wind?**

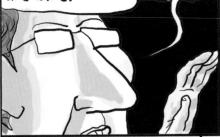

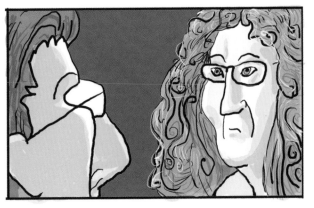

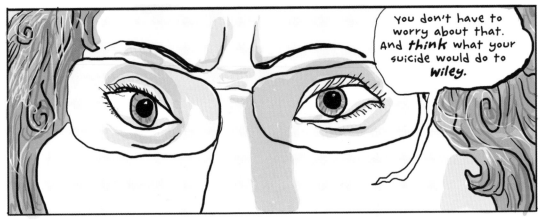

You don't have to worry about that. And **think** what your suicide would do to **wiley.**

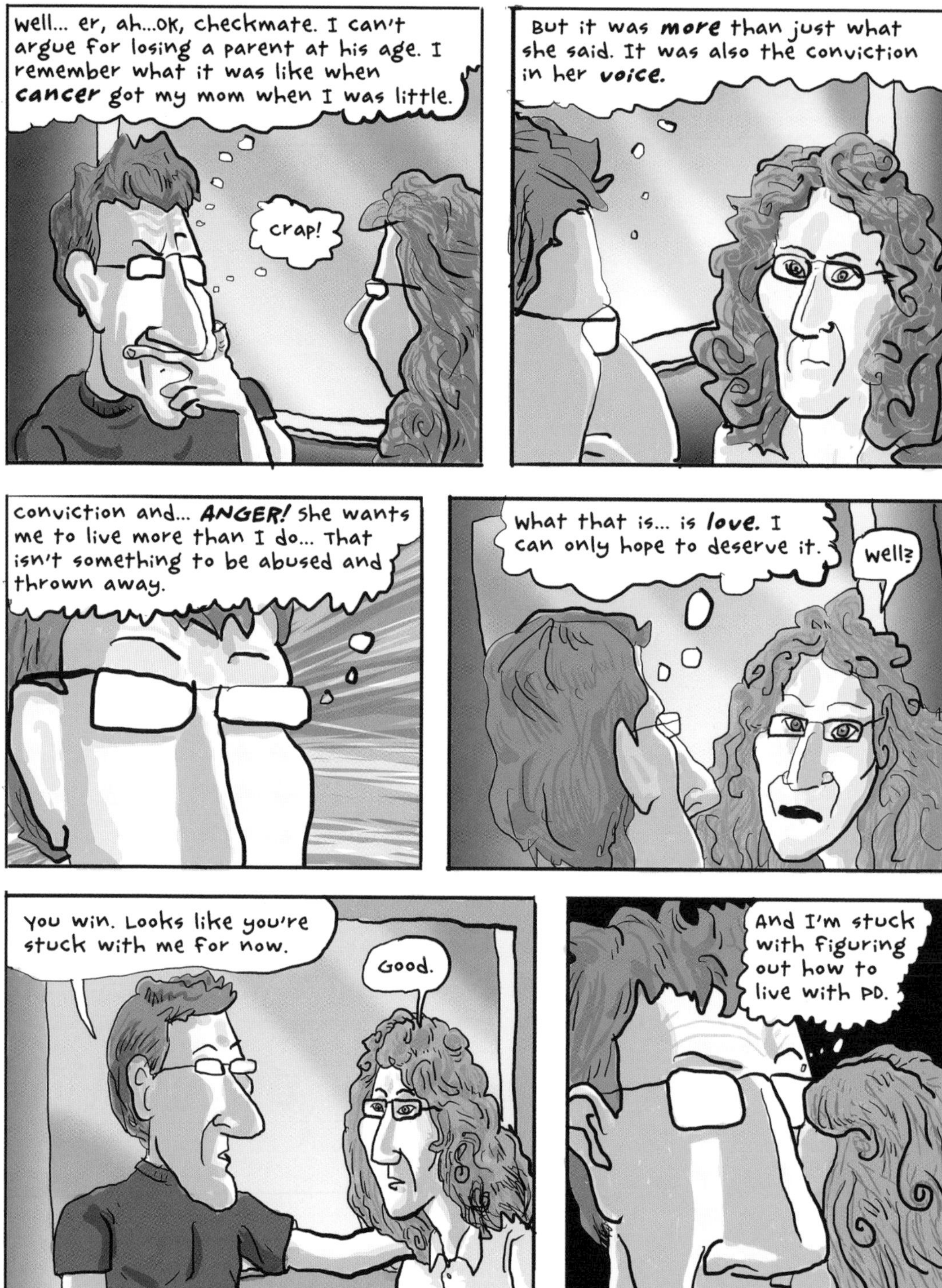
Well... er, ah...OK, checkmate. I can't argue for losing a parent at his age. I remember what it was like when **cancer** got my mom when I was little.
crap!
But it was **more** than just what she said. It was also the conviction in her **voice.**
conviction and... **ANGER!** She wants me to live more than I do... That isn't something to be abused and thrown away.
What that is... is **love.** I can only hope to deserve it.
Well?
You win. Looks like you're stuck with me for now.
Good.
And I'm stuck with figuring out how to live with PD.

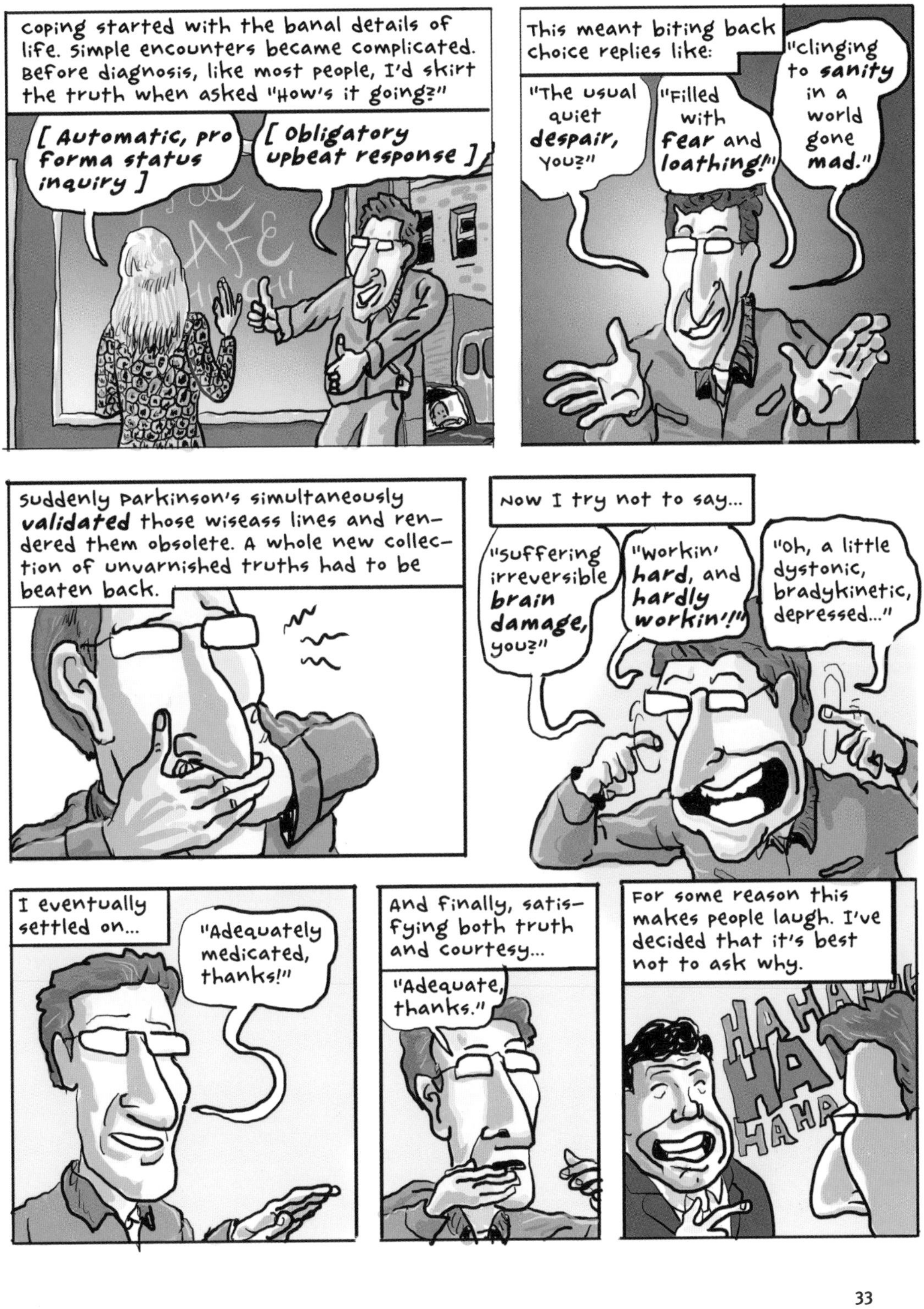
Coping started with the banal details of life. Simple encounters became complicated. Before diagnosis, like most people, I'd skirt the truth when asked "How's it going?"
[Automatic, pro forma status inquiry]
[Obligatory upbeat response]
This meant biting back choice replies like:
"The usual quiet despair, you?"
"Filled with fear and loathing!"
"Clinging to sanity in a world gone mad."
Suddenly Parkinson's simultaneously validated those wiseass lines and rendered them obsolete. A whole new collection of unvarnished truths had to be beaten back.
Now I try not to say...
"Suffering irreversible brain damage, you?"
"Workin' hard, and hardly workin'!"
"Oh, a little dystonic, bradykinetic, depressed..."
I eventually settled on...
"Adequately medicated, thanks!"
And finally, satisfying both truth and courtesy...
"Adequate, thanks."
For some reason this makes people laugh. I've decided that it's best not to ask why.
HAHAHAHA
HA
HA
HAHA

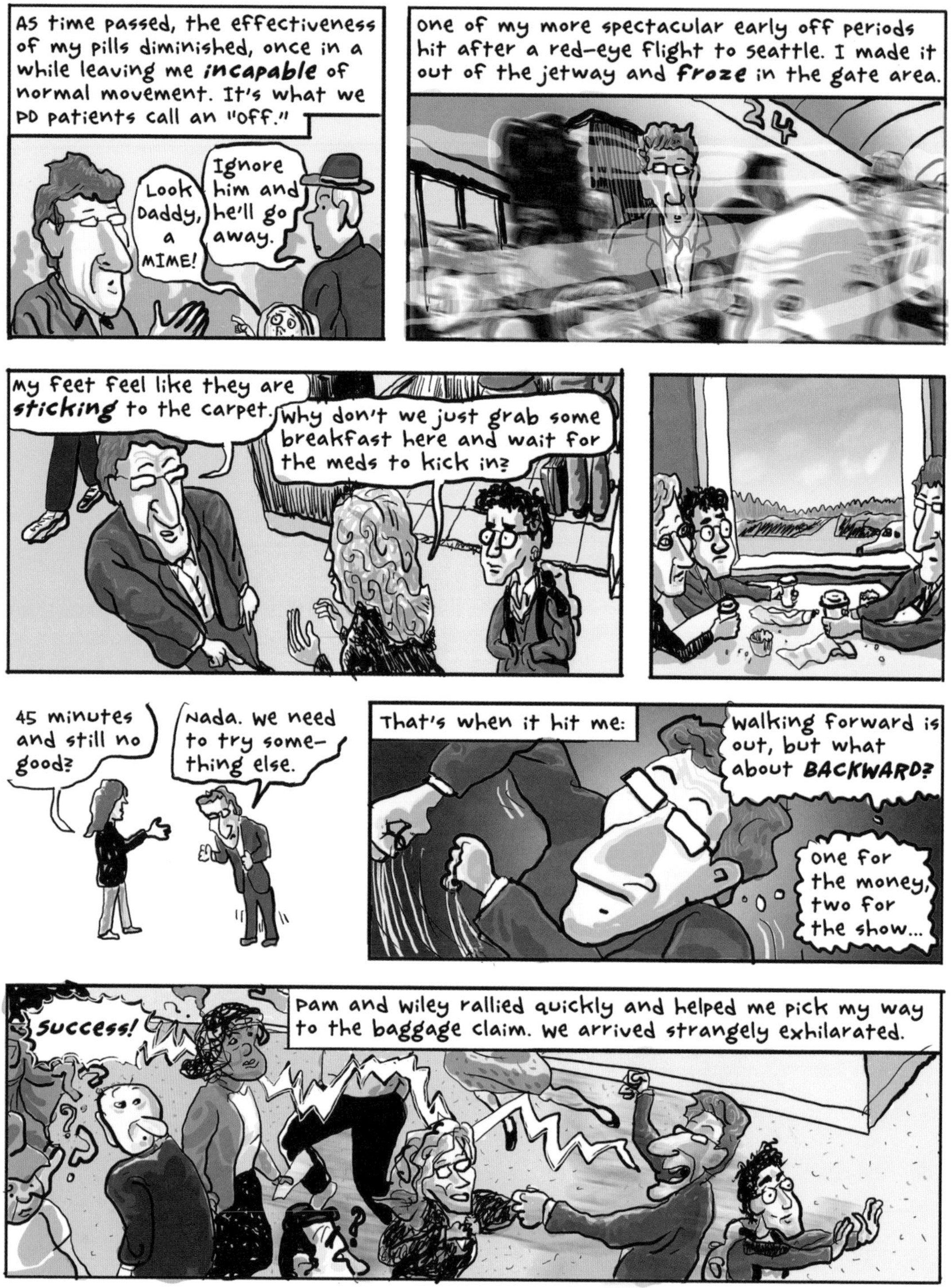
As time passed, the effectiveness of my pills diminished, once in a while leaving me *incapable* of normal movement. It's what we PD patients call an "off."
Look Daddy, a MIME!
Ignore him and he'll go away.
One of my more spectacular early off periods hit after a red-eye flight to Seattle. I made it out of the jetway and *froze* in the gate area.
24
My feet feel like they are *sticking* to the carpet.
Why don't we just grab some breakfast here and wait for the meds to kick in?
45 minutes and still no good?
Nada. We need to try something else.
That's when it hit me:
Walking forward is out, but what about **BACKWARD?**
One for the money, two for the show...
SUCCESS!
Pam and Wiley rallied quickly and helped me pick my way to the baggage claim. We arrived strangely exhilarated.

Walk This Way, strategies to keep you moving

NOTE: If your balance is shot, these may not be for you.

PD has halted me countless times. Here are some ways I found over the years to get moving. Why do they work? I don't know. I just chalk it up to the malicious whimsy of this strange affliction.

1: Walk Backward. Use in open areas that present minimal danger of falling over unseen objects. Get someone to spot you.

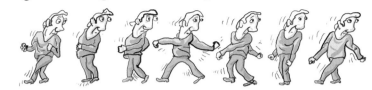

2: Throwing Toes. Have a nimble companion start you by placing a toe in front of yours to step over.

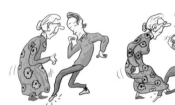

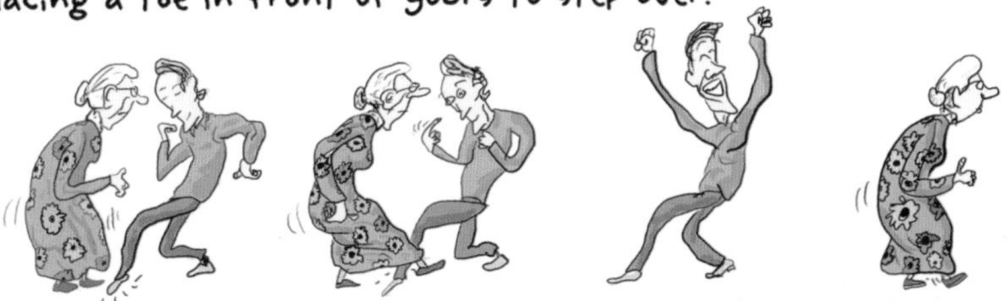

3: Walk pigeon-toed. While stranded with nobody to throw me a toe, I thought, "Why not just step over my own toe?" Yes, it looks stupid. So does standing frozen like a wax replica of yourself.

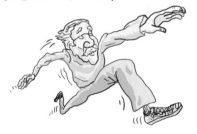

4: The Straddle Step. If there is a curb handy, try walking with one foot on the curb and the other on the adjacent lower surface.

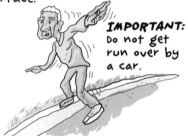

IMPORTANT: Do not get run over by a car.

5: The Flying Leap. Sometimes what is needed is a dramatic move. Often when I cannot walk, I can skip.

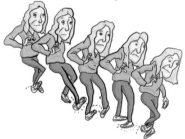

6: Ragkicker's Dream. Drop a soft object on the floor (I use a glasses cleaning cloth). Now kick, and follow, kick and follow...

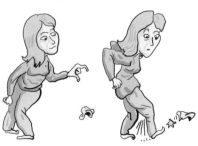

35

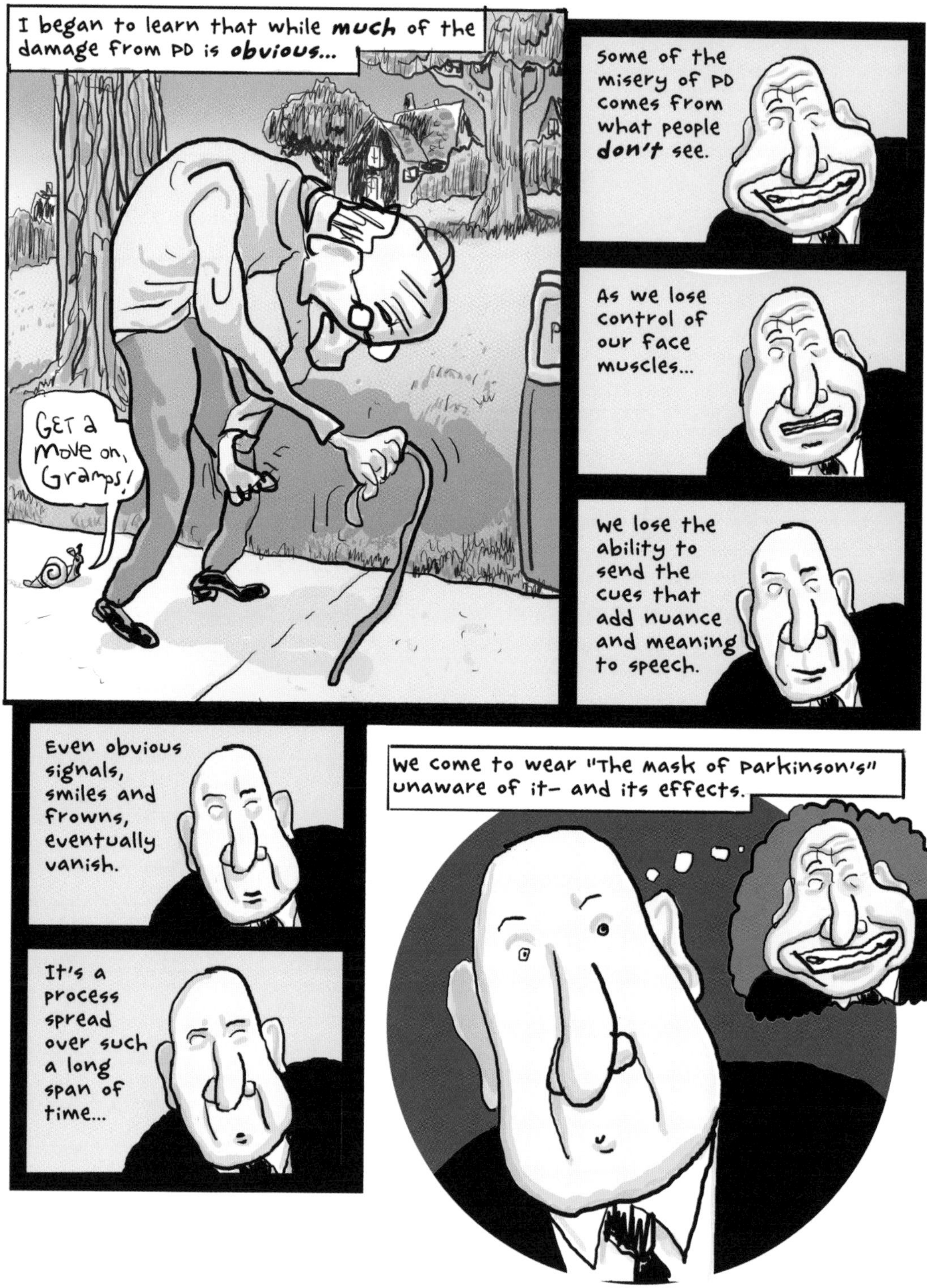
I began to learn that while **much** of the damage from PD is **obvious...**
GET a move on, Gramps!
Some of the misery of PD comes from what people **don't** see.
As we lose control of our face muscles...
We lose the ability to send the cues that add nuance and meaning to speech.
Even obvious signals, smiles and frowns, eventually vanish.
It's a process spread over such a long span of time...
We come to wear "The mask of Parkinson's" unaware of it— and its effects.

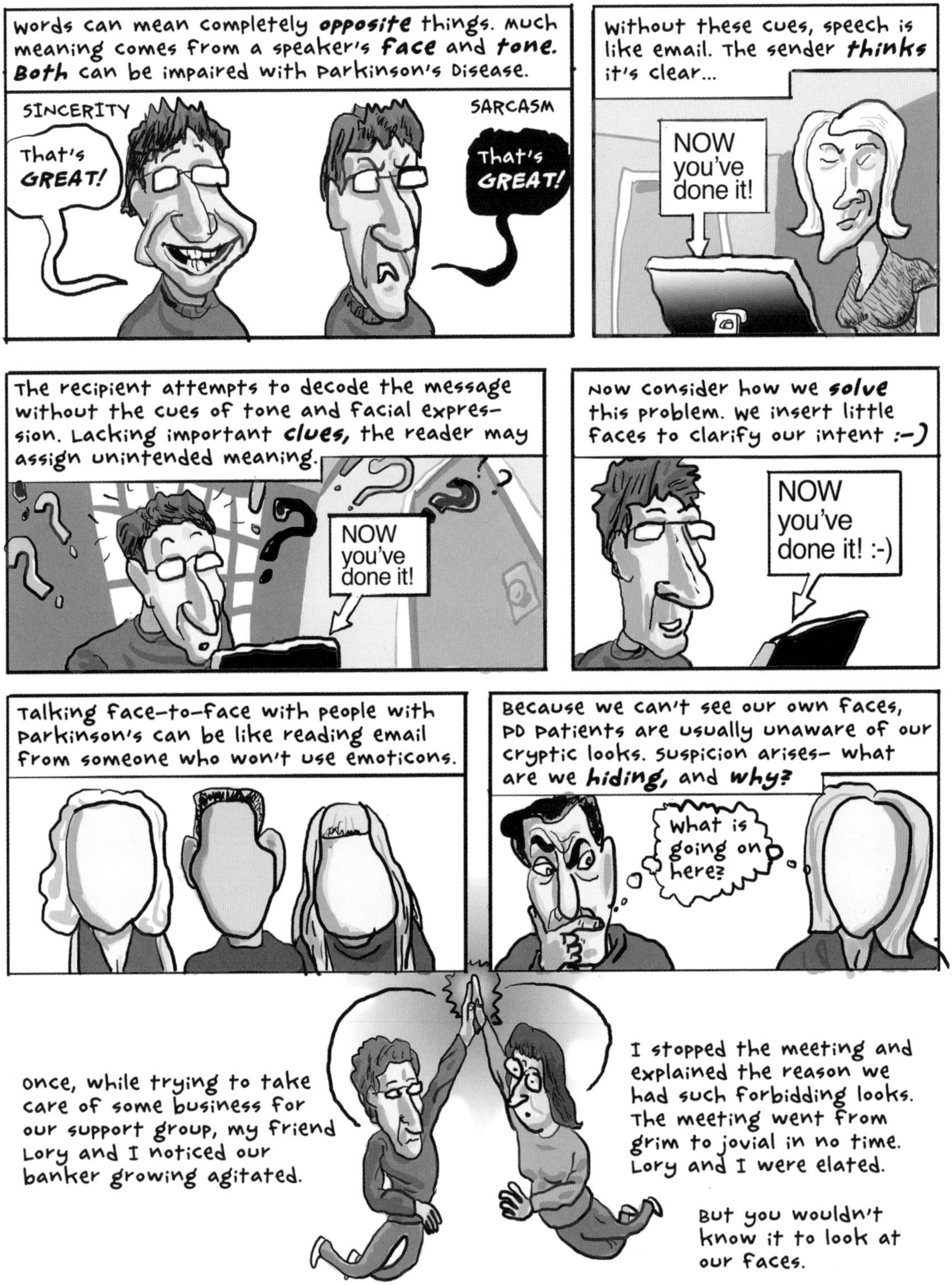

Words can mean completely **opposite** things. Much meaning comes from a speaker's **face** and **tone.** **Both** can be impaired with Parkinson's Disease.
SINCERITY
That's GREAT!
SARCASM
That's GREAT!
Without these cues, speech is like email. The sender **thinks** it's clear...
NOW you've done it!
The recipient attempts to decode the message without the cues of tone and facial expression. Lacking important **clues,** the reader may assign unintended meaning.
NOW you've done it!
Now consider how we **solve** this problem. We insert little faces to clarify our intent :–)
NOW you've done it! :-)
Talking face-to-face with people with Parkinson's can be like reading email from someone who won't use emoticons.
Because we can't see our own faces, PD patients are usually unaware of our cryptic looks. Suspicion arises– what are we **hiding,** and **why?**
What is going on here?
Once, while trying to take care of some business for our support group, my friend Lory and I noticed our banker growing agitated.
I stopped the meeting and explained the reason we had such forbidding looks. The meeting went from grim to jovial in no time. Lory and I were elated.
But you wouldn't know it to look at our faces.

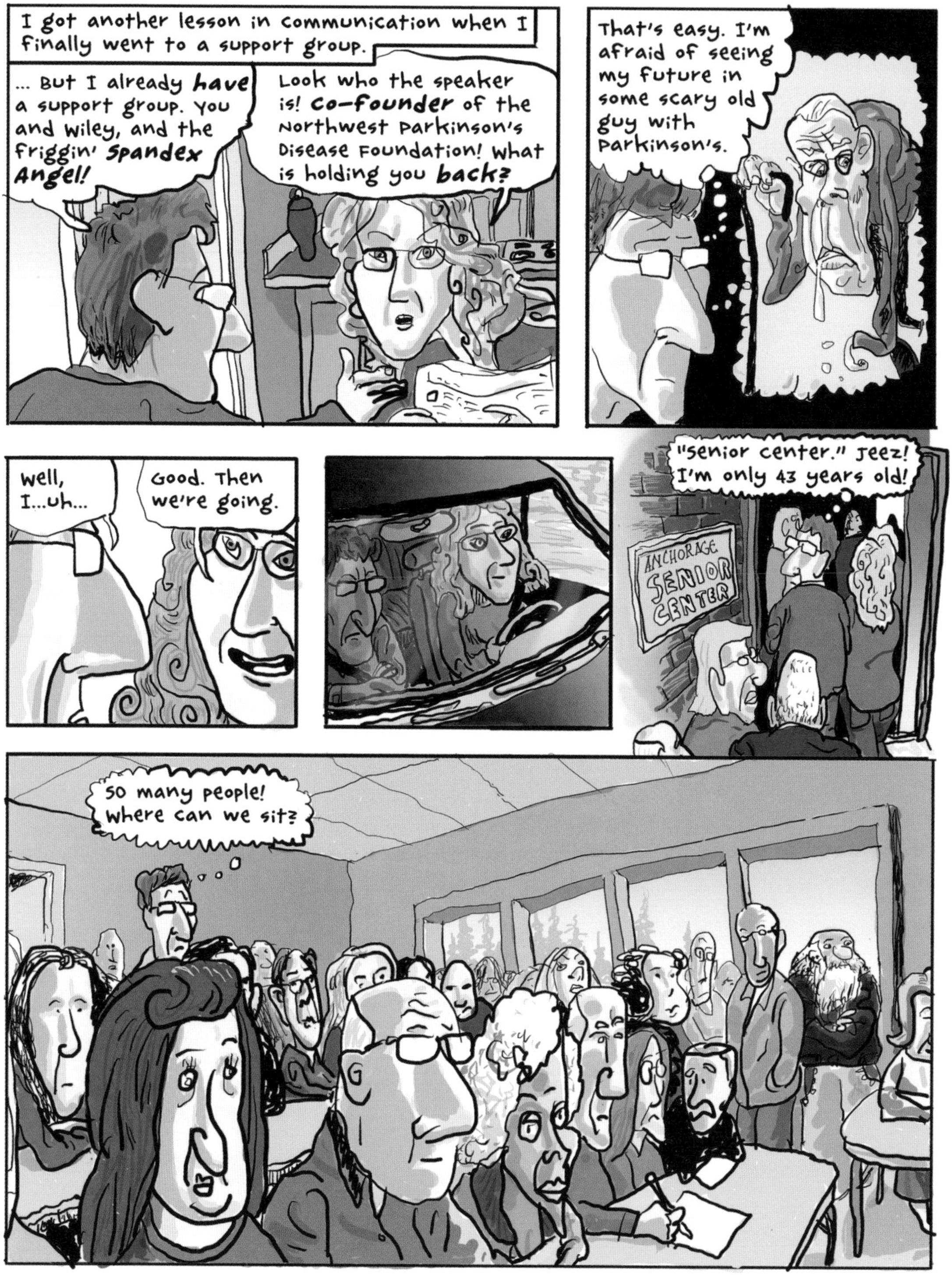
I got another lesson in communication when I finally went to a support group.
... But I already **have** a support group. You and Wiley, and the friggin' **Spandex Angel!**
Look who the speaker is! **Co-founder** of the Northwest Parkinson's Disease Foundation! What is holding you **back?**
That's easy. I'm afraid of seeing my future in some scary old guy with Parkinson's.
Well, I...uh...
Good. Then we're going.
"Senior center." Jeez! I'm only 43 years old!
ANCHORAGE SENIOR CENTER
So many people! Where can we sit?

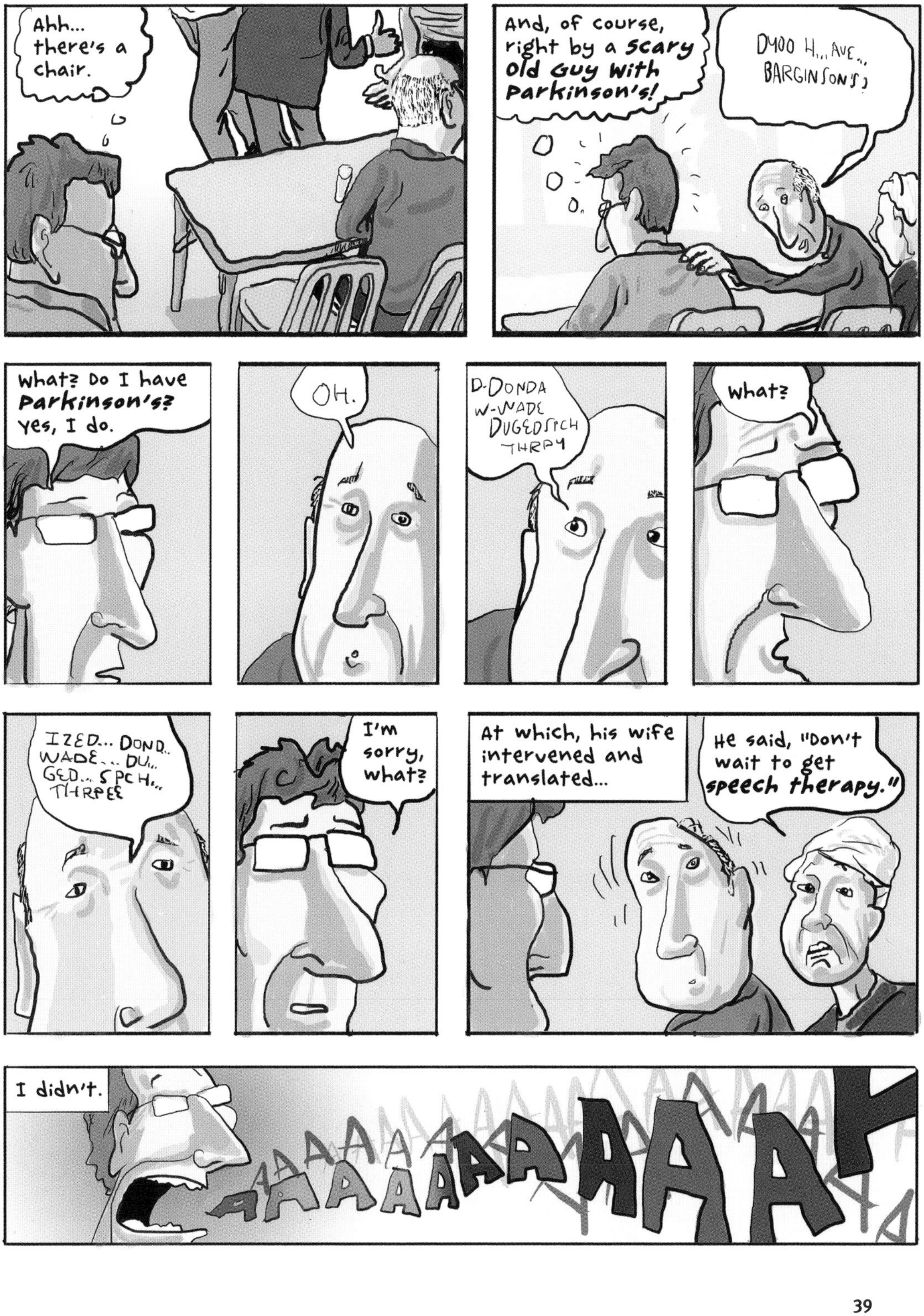
Ahh... there's a chair.
And, of course, right by a scary old guy with Parkinson's!
DYOO H... AVE... BARGINSON'S?
What? Do I have Parkinson's? Yes, I do.
OH.
D-DONDA W-WADE DUGEDSPCH THRPY
What?
IZED... DOND... WADE... DU... GED... SPCH... THRPEE
I'm sorry, what?
At which, his wife intervened and translated...
He said, "Don't wait to get speech therapy."
I didn't.
AAAAAAAAAAAAAAAH

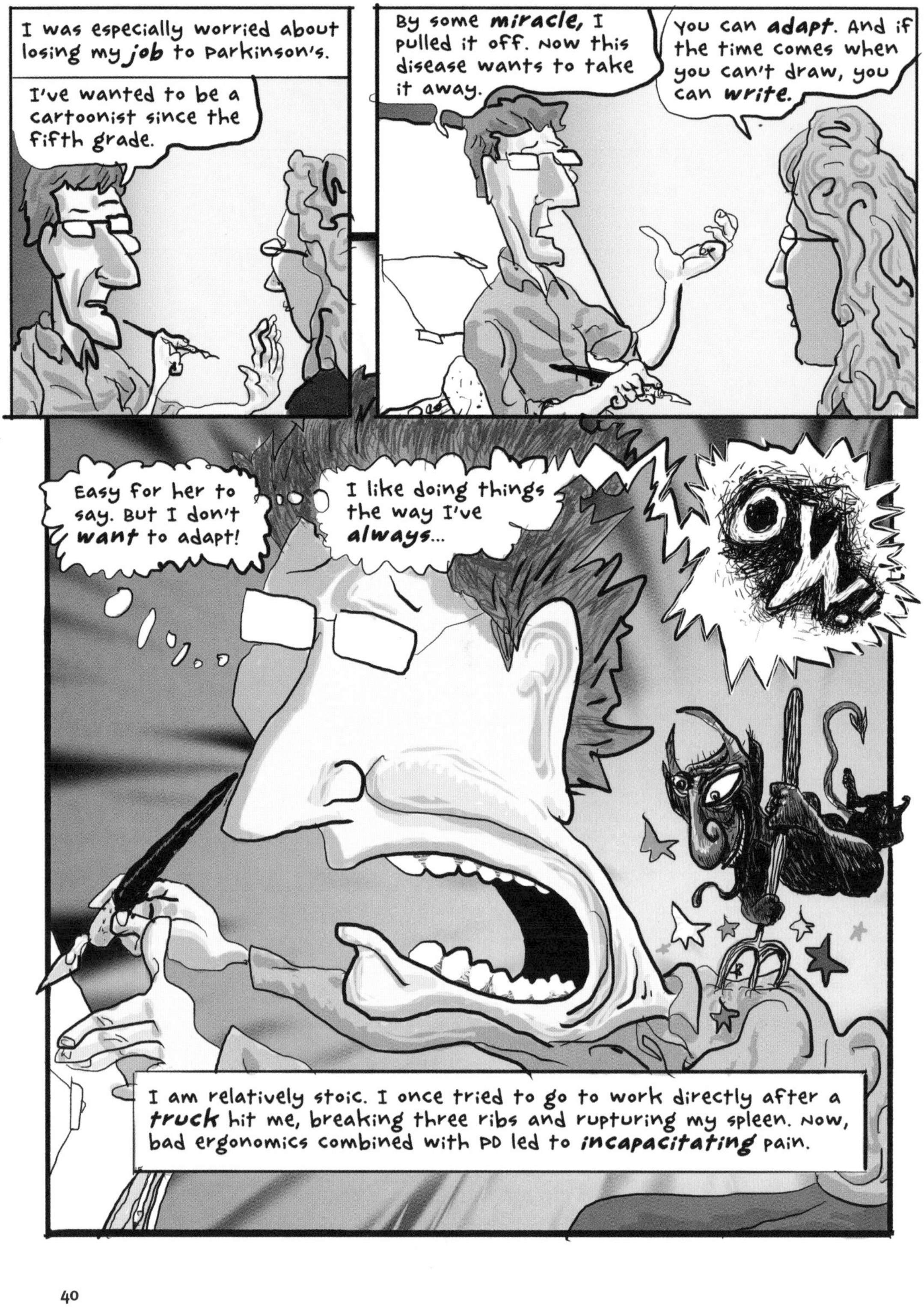
I was especially worried about losing my job to Parkinson's.
I've wanted to be a cartoonist since the fifth grade.
By some miracle, I pulled it off. Now this disease wants to take it away.
You can adapt. And if the time comes when you can't draw, you can write.
Easy for her to say. But I don't want to adapt!
I like doing things the way I've always...
OW!
I am relatively stoic. I once tried to go to work directly after a truck hit me, breaking three ribs and rupturing my spleen. Now, bad ergonomics combined with PD led to incapacitating pain.

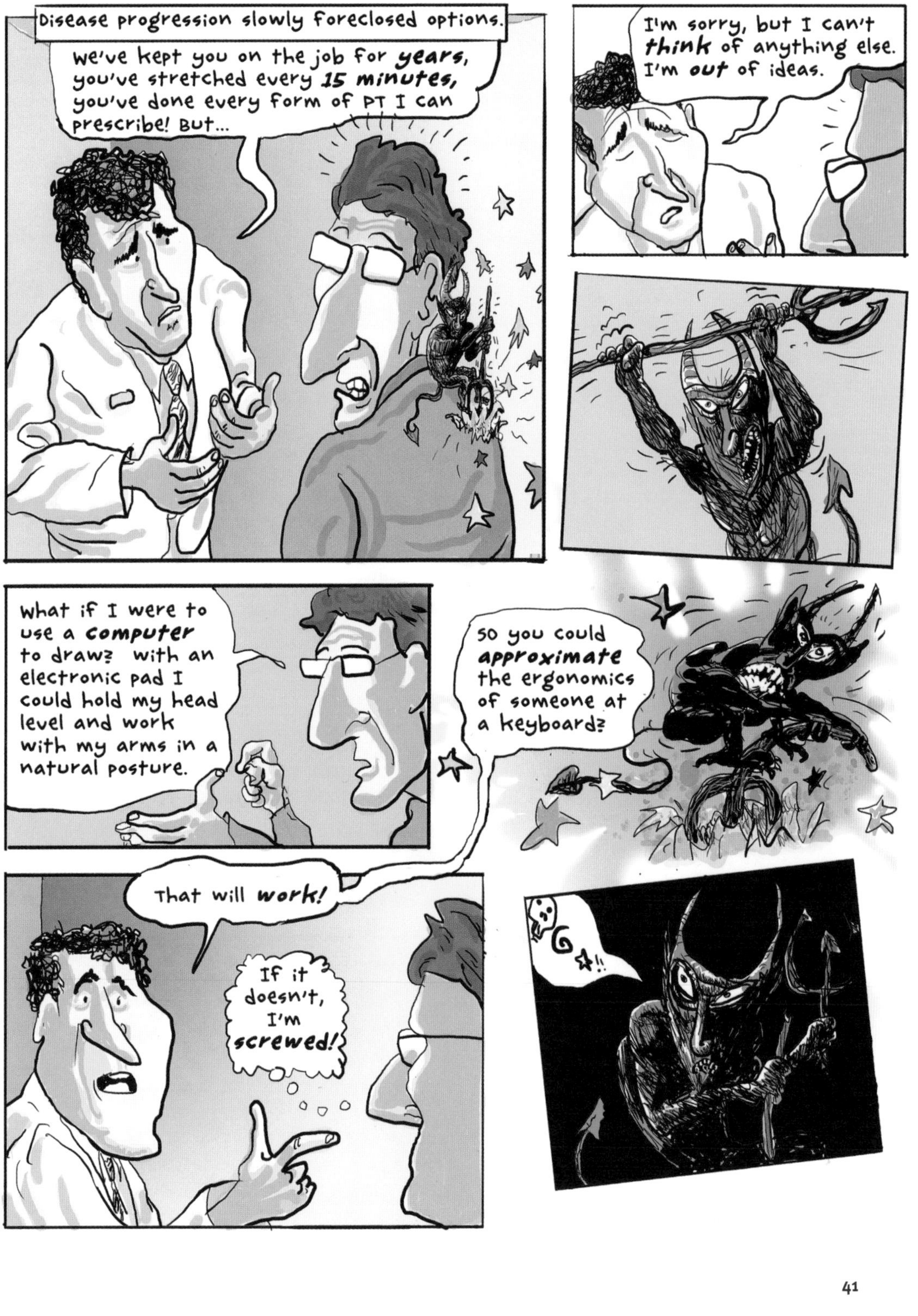
Disease progression slowly foreclosed options.
We've kept you on the job for years, you've stretched every 15 minutes, you've done every form of PT I can prescribe! But...
I'm sorry, but I can't think of anything else. I'm out of ideas.
What if I were to use a computer to draw? with an electronic pad I could hold my head level and work with my arms in a natural posture.
So you could approximate the ergonomics of someone at a keyboard?
That will work!
If it doesn't, I'm screwed!

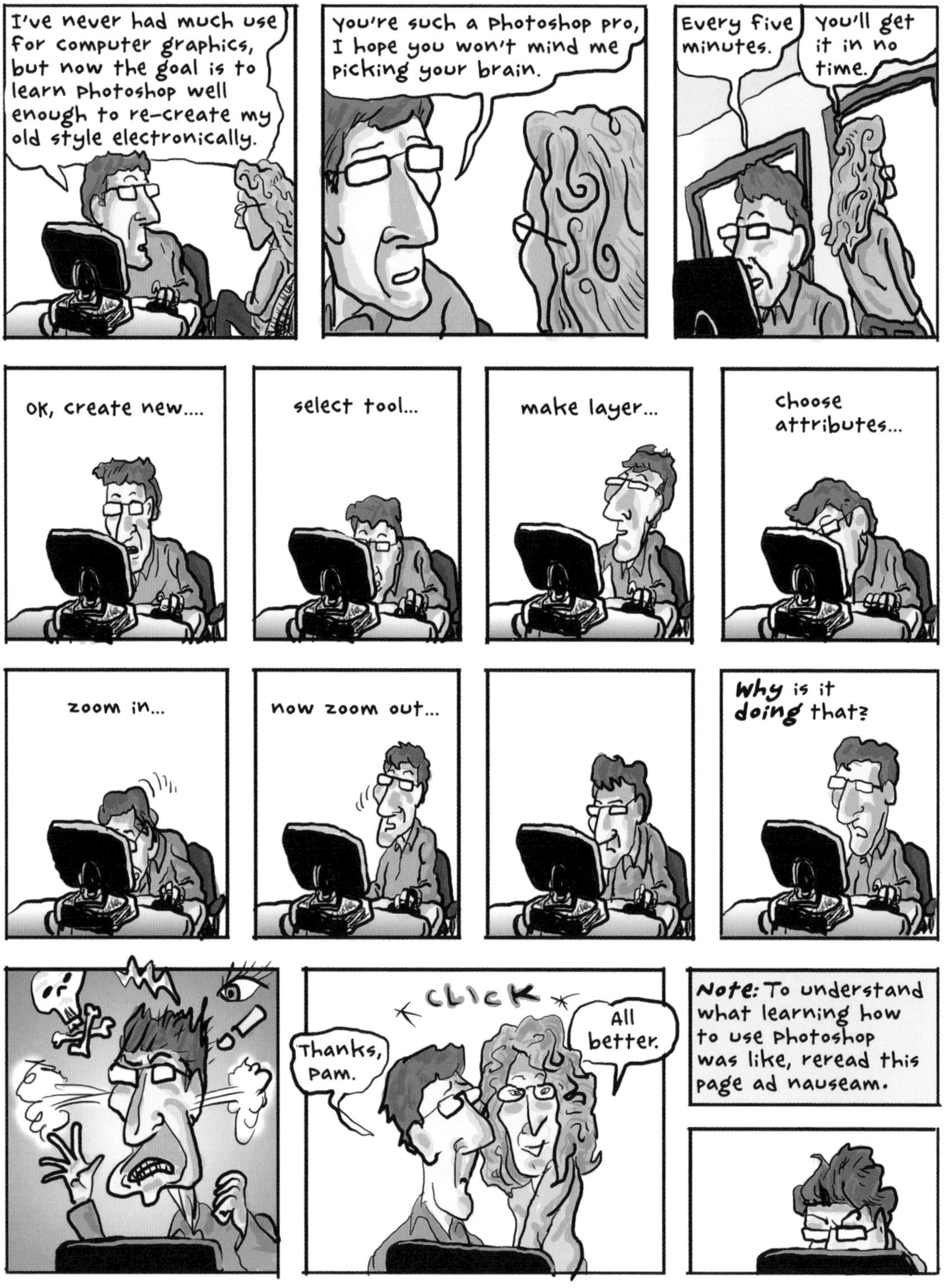
I've never had much use for computer graphics, but now the goal is to learn Photoshop well enough to re-create my old style electronically.
You're such a Photoshop pro, I hope you won't mind me picking your brain.
Every five minutes.
You'll get it in no time.
OK, create new....
select tool...
make layer...
choose attributes...
zoom in...
now zoom out...
Why is it **doing** that?
CLICK
Thanks, Pam.
All better.
Note: To understand what learning how to use Photoshop was like, reread this page ad nauseam.

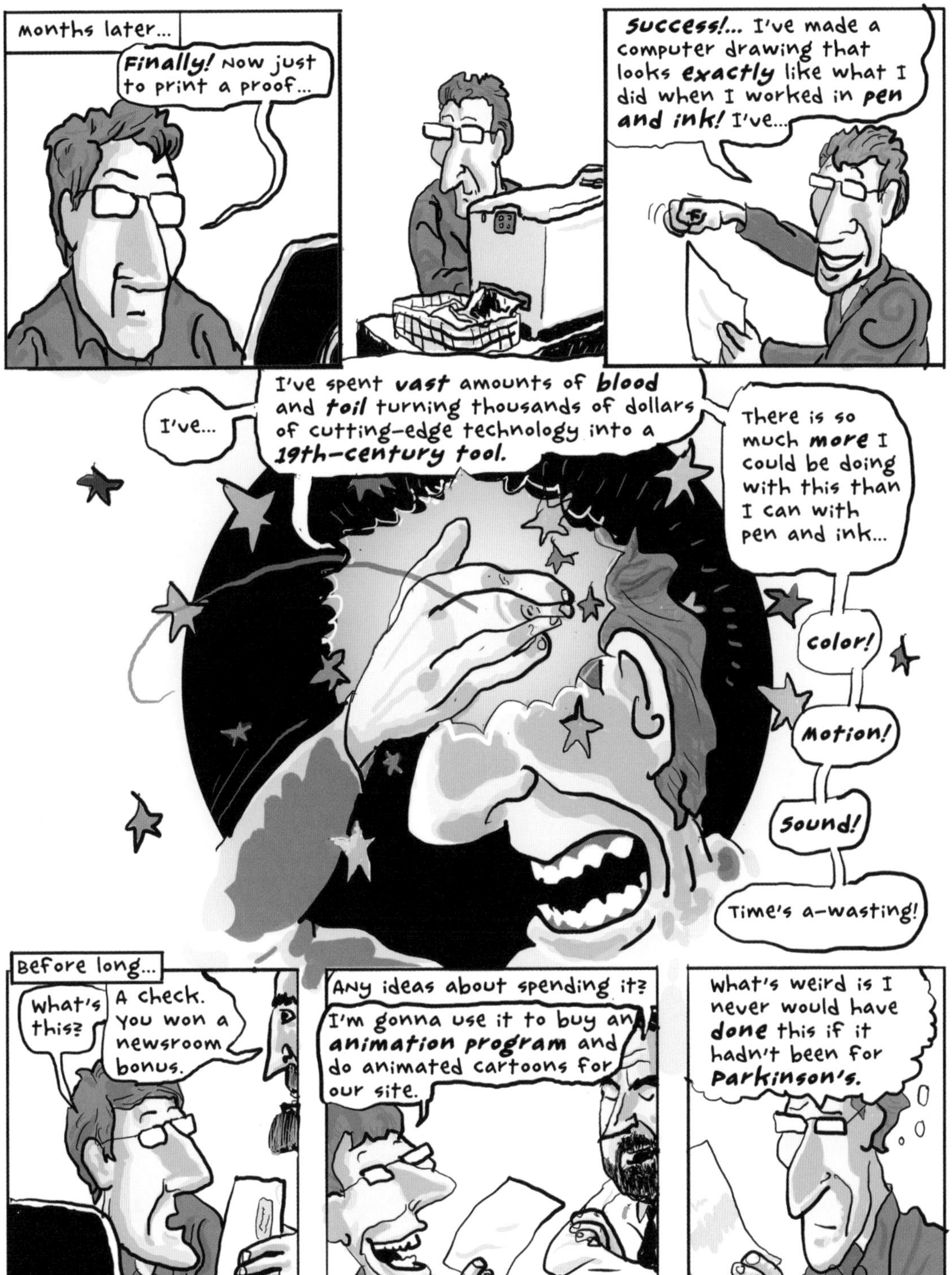

months later...
Finally! Now just to print a proof...
Success!... I've made a computer drawing that looks exactly like what I did when I worked in pen and ink! I've...
I've...
I've spent vast amounts of blood and toil turning thousands of dollars of cutting-edge technology into a 19th-century tool.
There is so much more I could be doing with this than I can with pen and ink...
color!
Motion!
Sound!
Time's a-wasting!
Before long...
What's this?
A check. You won a newsroom bonus.
Any ideas about spending it?
I'm gonna use it to buy an animation program and do animated cartoons for our site.
What's weird is I never would have done this if it hadn't been for Parkinson's.

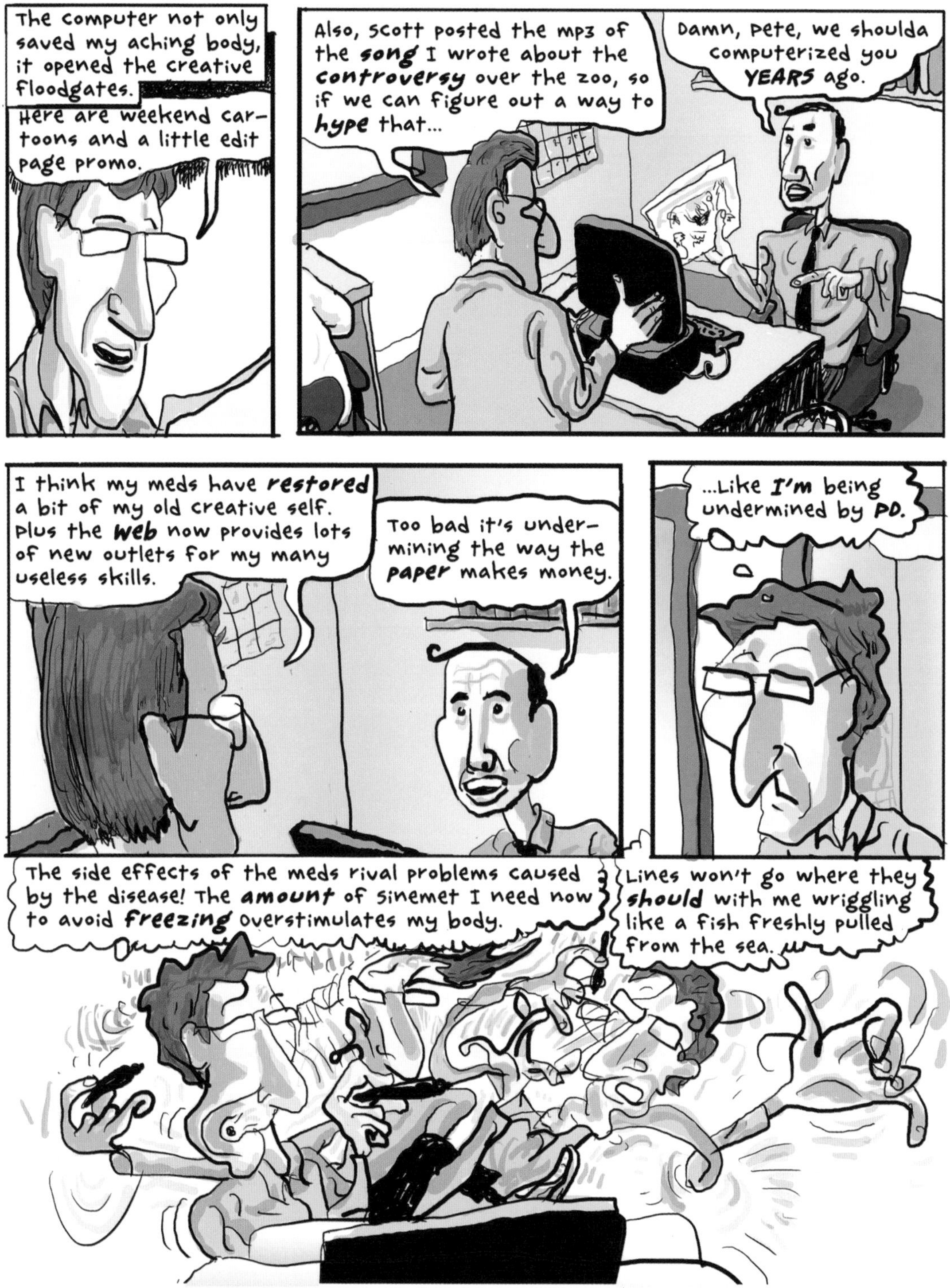
The computer not only saved my aching body, it opened the creative floodgates.
Here are weekend cartoons and a little edit page promo.
Also, Scott posted the mp3 of the song I wrote about the controversy over the zoo, so if we can figure out a way to hype that...
Damn, Pete, we shoulda computerized you YEARS ago.
I think my meds have restored a bit of my old creative self. Plus the web now provides lots of new outlets for my many useless skills.
Too bad it's undermining the way the paper makes money.
...Like I'm being undermined by PD.
The side effects of the meds rival problems caused by the disease! The amount of sinemet I need now to avoid freezing overstimulates my body.
Lines won't go where they should with me wriggling like a fish freshly pulled from the sea.

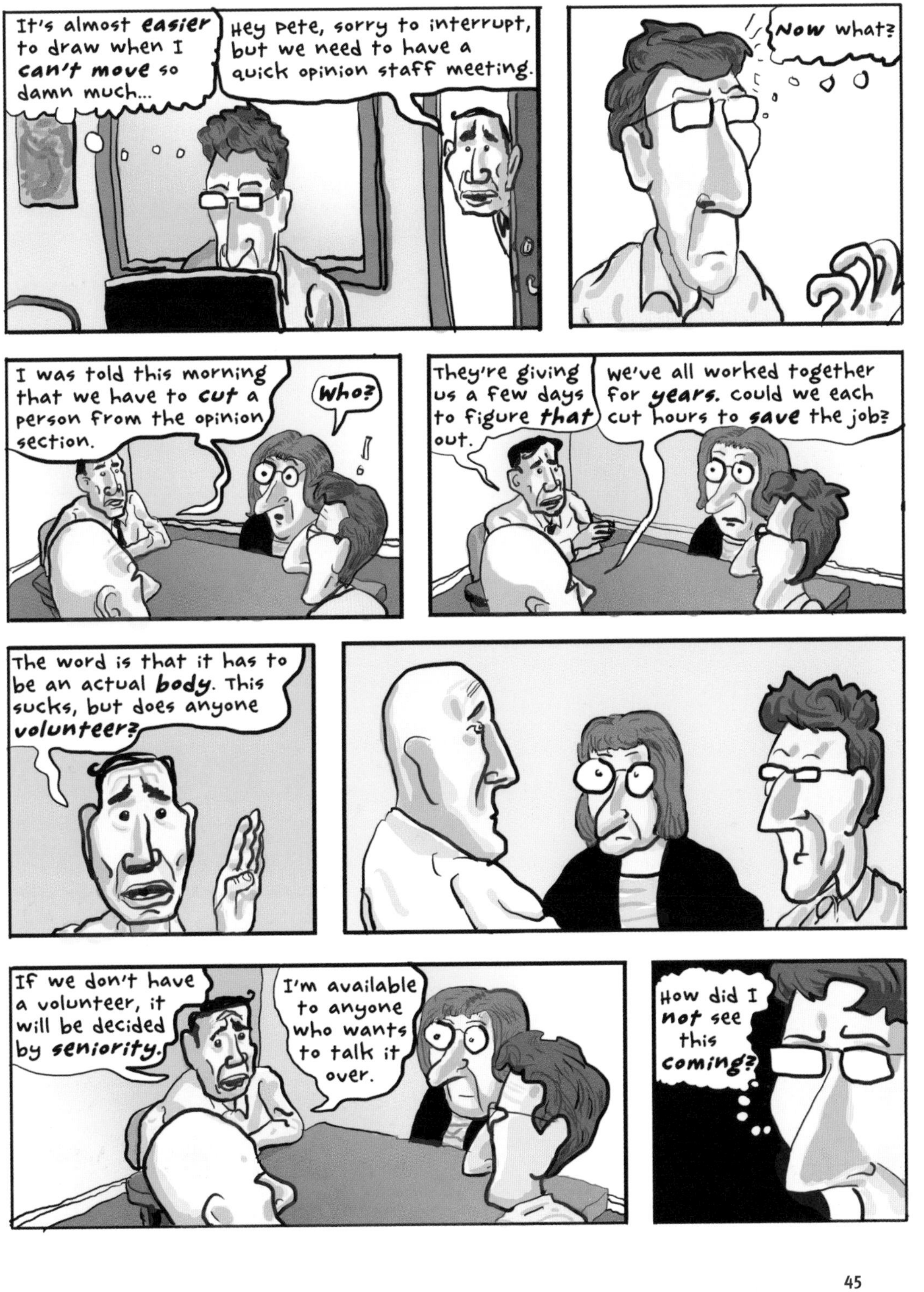
It's almost easier to draw when I can't move so damn much...
Hey Pete, sorry to interrupt, but we need to have a quick opinion staff meeting.
Now what?
I was told this morning that we have to cut a person from the opinion section.
Who?
They're giving us a few days to figure that out.
We've all worked together for years. Could we each cut hours to save the job?
The word is that it has to be an actual body. This sucks, but does anyone volunteer?
If we don't have a volunteer, it will be decided by seniority.
I'm available to anyone who wants to talk it over.
How did I not see this coming?

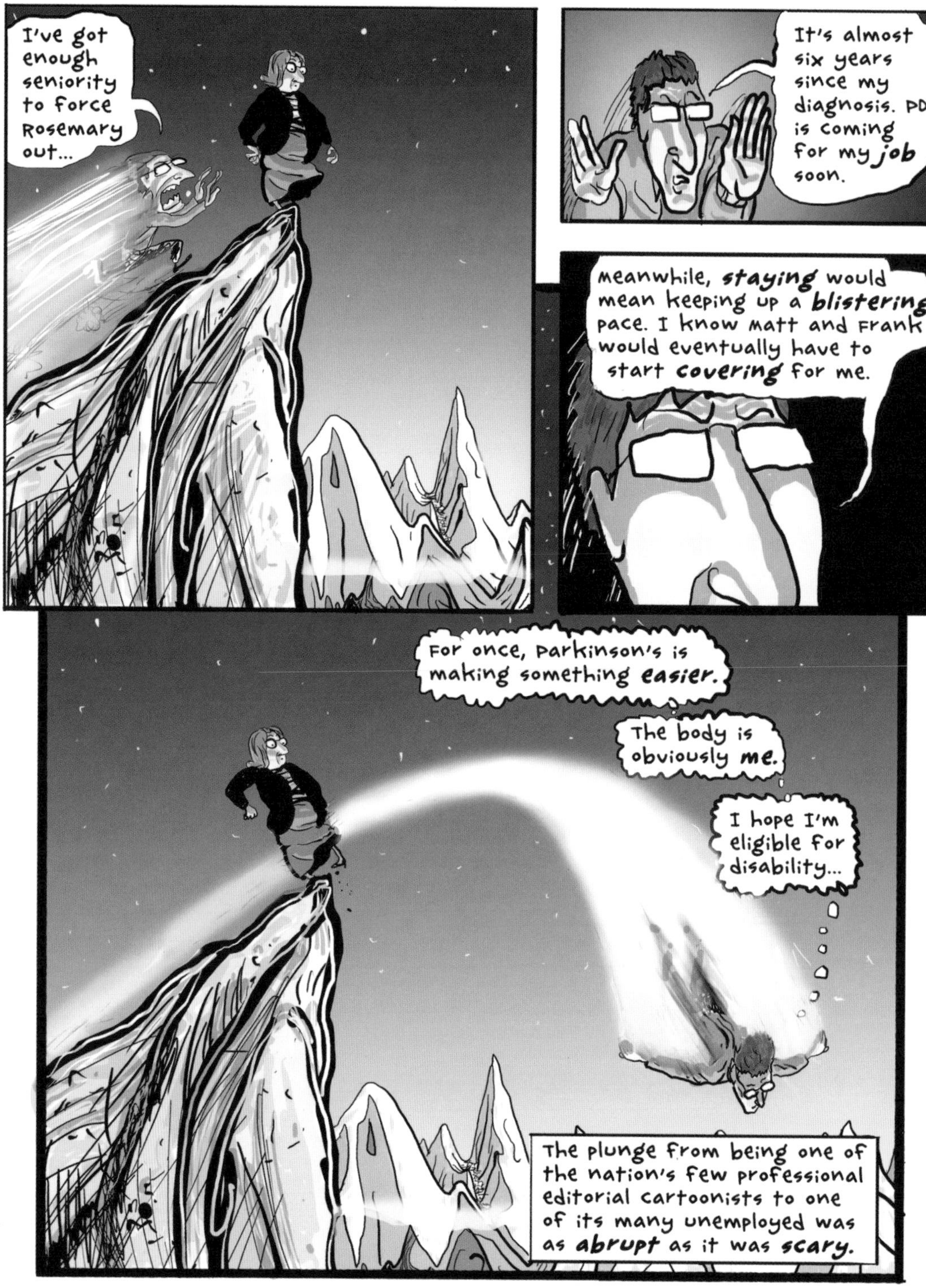

I've got enough seniority to force Rosemary out...
It's almost six years since my diagnosis. PD is coming for my job soon.
Meanwhile, staying would mean keeping up a blistering pace. I know Matt and Frank would eventually have to start covering for me.
For once, Parkinson's is making something easier.
The body is obviously me.
I hope I'm eligible for disability...
The plunge from being one of the nation's few professional editorial cartoonists to one of its many unemployed was as abrupt as it was scary.

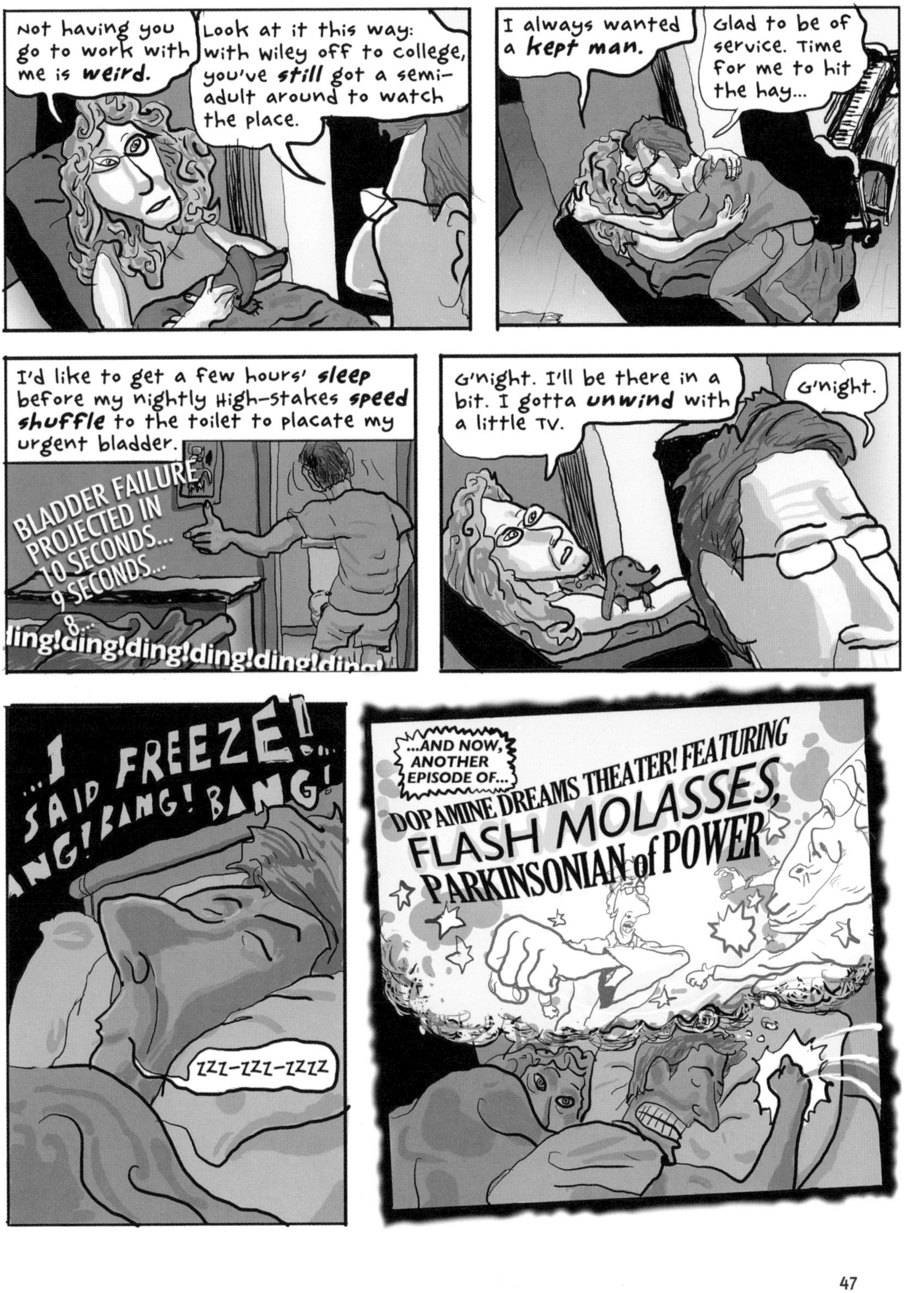
Not having you go to work with me is weird.
Look at it this way: with Wiley off to college, you've still got a semi-adult around to watch the place.
I always wanted a kept man.
Glad to be of service. Time for me to hit the hay...
I'd like to get a few hours' sleep before my nightly High-stakes speed shuffle to the toilet to placate my urgent bladder.
BLADDER FAILURE PROJECTED IN 10 SECONDS... 9 SECONDS... 8...
ding!ding!ding!ding!ding!ding!
G'night. I'll be there in a bit. I gotta unwind with a little TV.
G'night.
...I SAID FREEZE!...
BANG! BANG! BANG!
ZZZ-ZZZ-ZZZZ
...AND NOW, ANOTHER EPISODE OF...
DOPAMINE DREAMS THEATER! FEATURING
FLASH MOLASSES, PARKINSONIAN of POWER

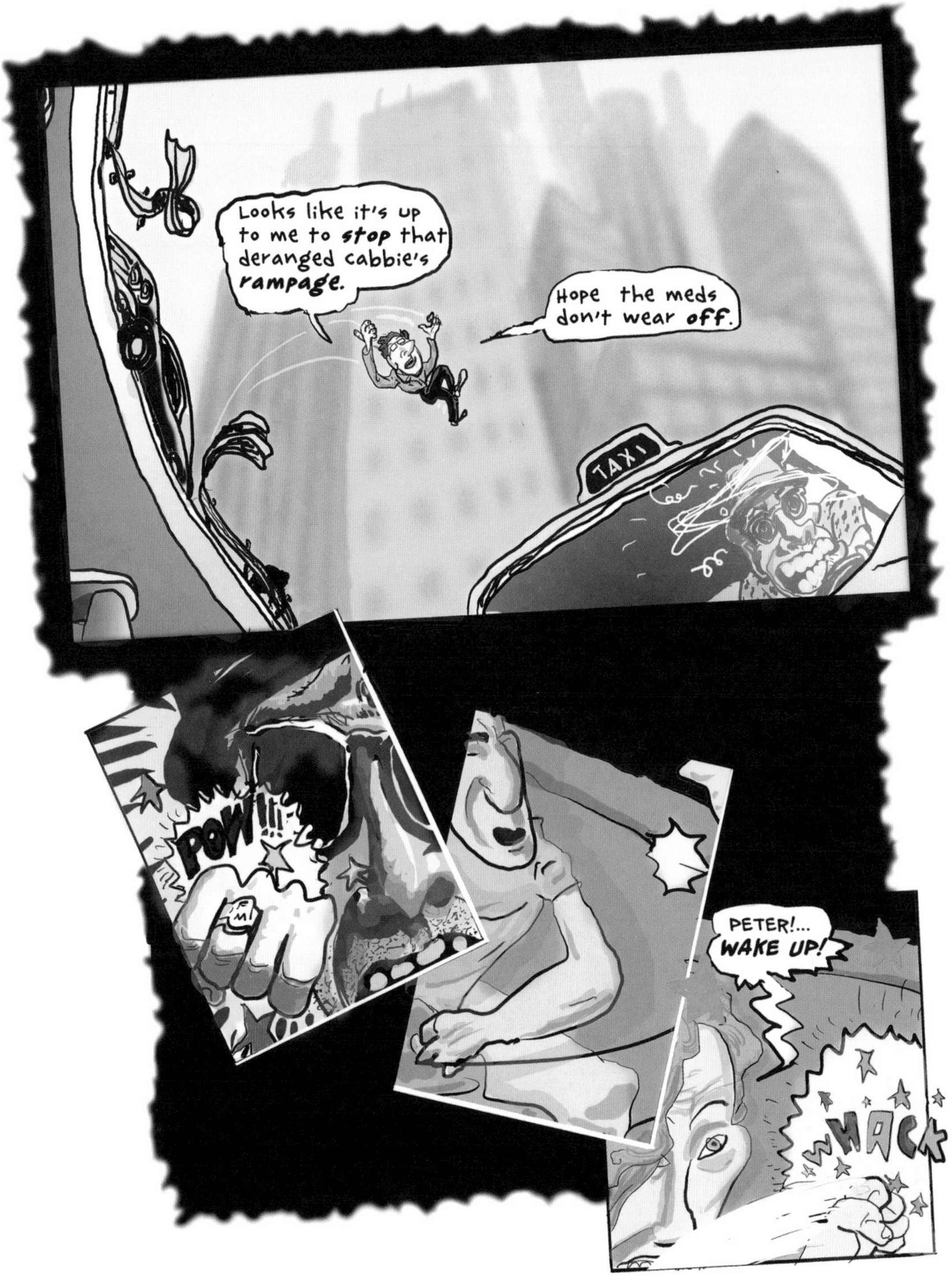
Looks like it's up to me to stop that deranged cabbie's rampage.
Hope the meds don't wear off.
TAXI
POW!!!
PETER!... WAKE UP!
WHACK

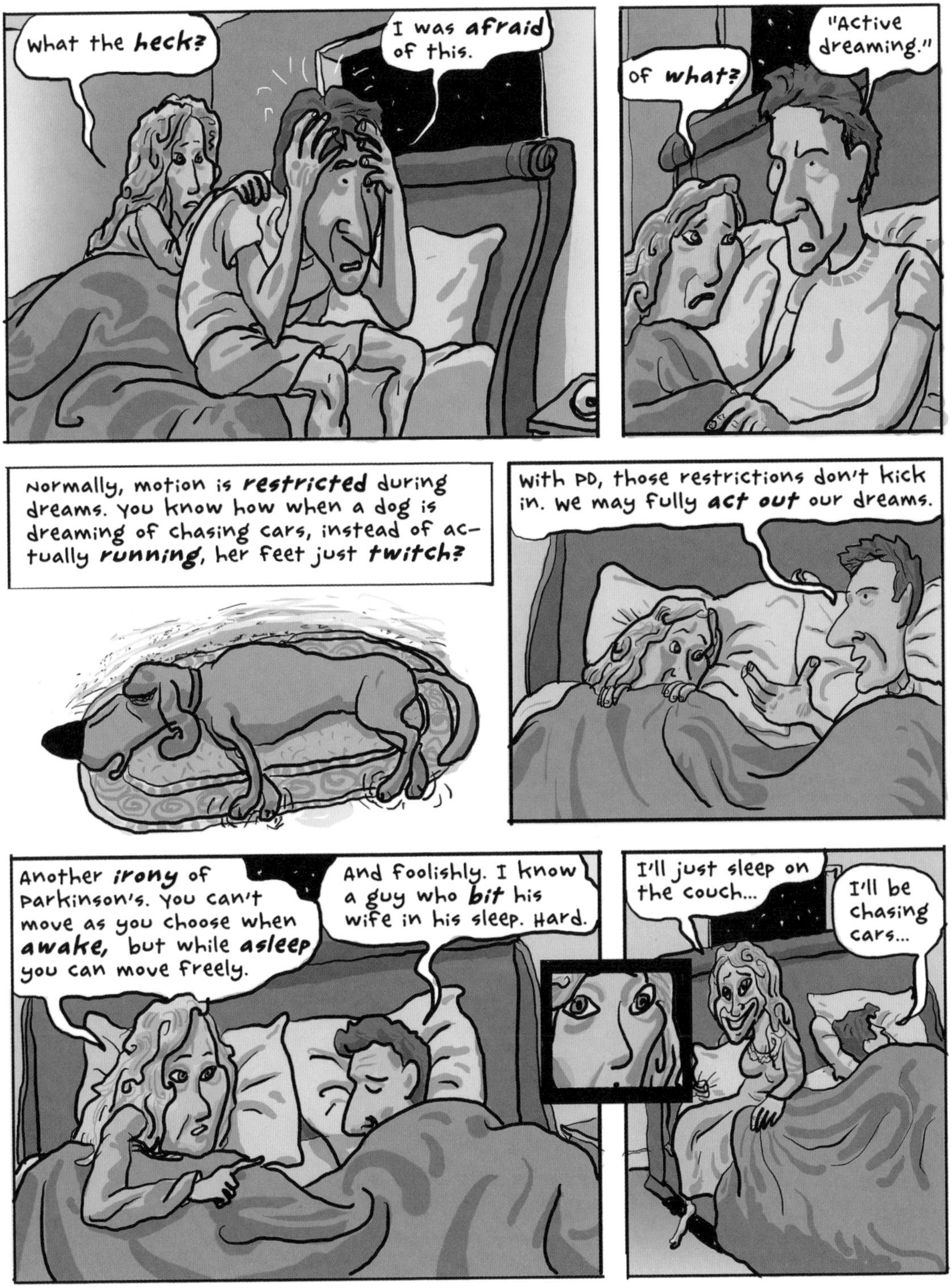
What the heck?
I was afraid of this.
Of what?
"Active dreaming."
Normally, motion is restricted during dreams. You know how when a dog is dreaming of chasing cars, instead of actually running, her feet just twitch?
With PD, those restrictions don't kick in. We may fully act out our dreams.
Another irony of Parkinson's. You can't move as you choose when awake, but while asleep you can move freely.
And foolishly. I know a guy who bit his wife in his sleep. Hard.
I'll just sleep on the couch...
I'll be chasing cars...

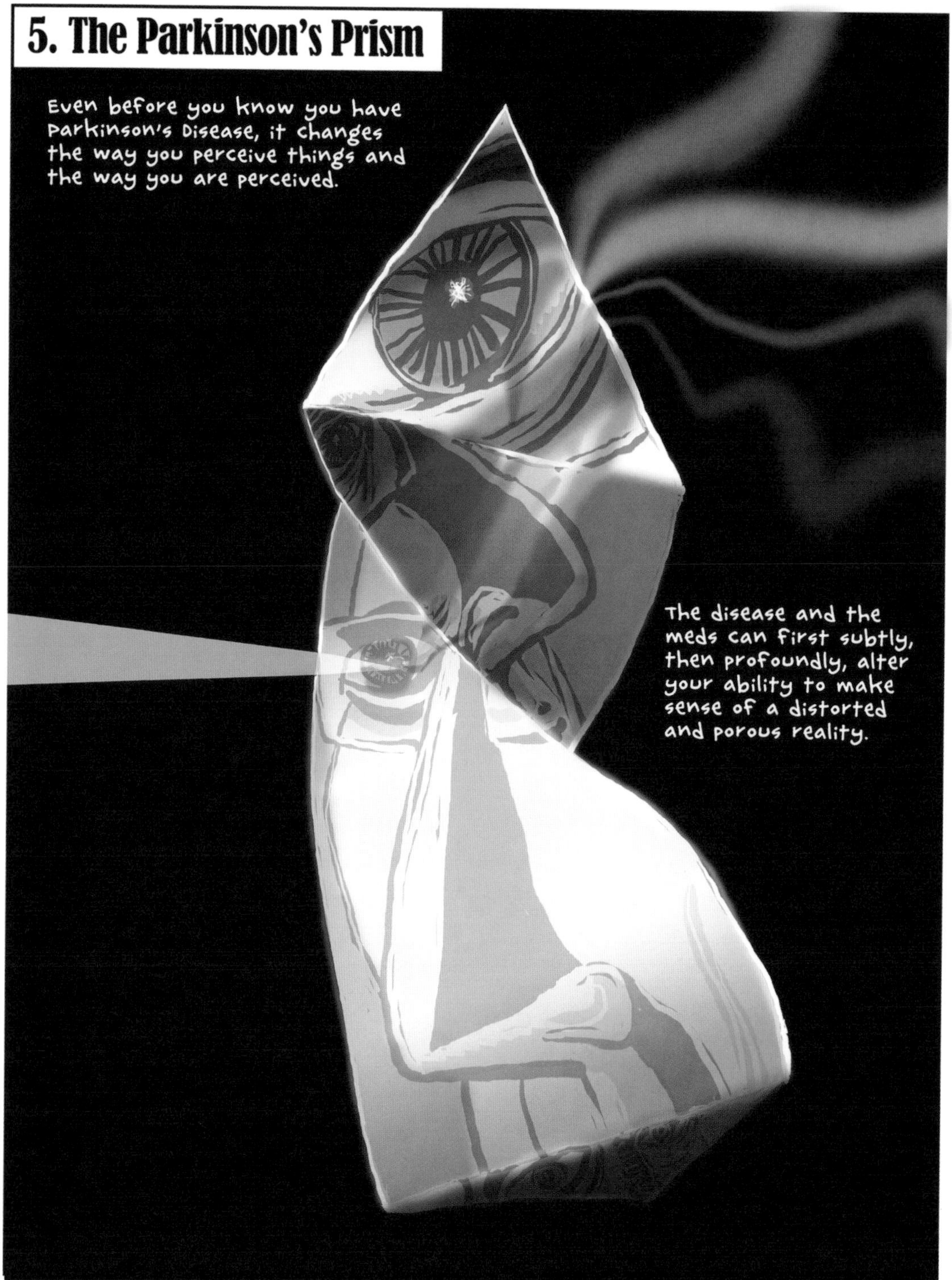
5. The Parkinson's Prism
Even before you know you have Parkinson's Disease, it changes the way you perceive things and the way you are perceived.
The disease and the meds can first subtly, then profoundly, alter your ability to make sense of a distorted and porous reality.

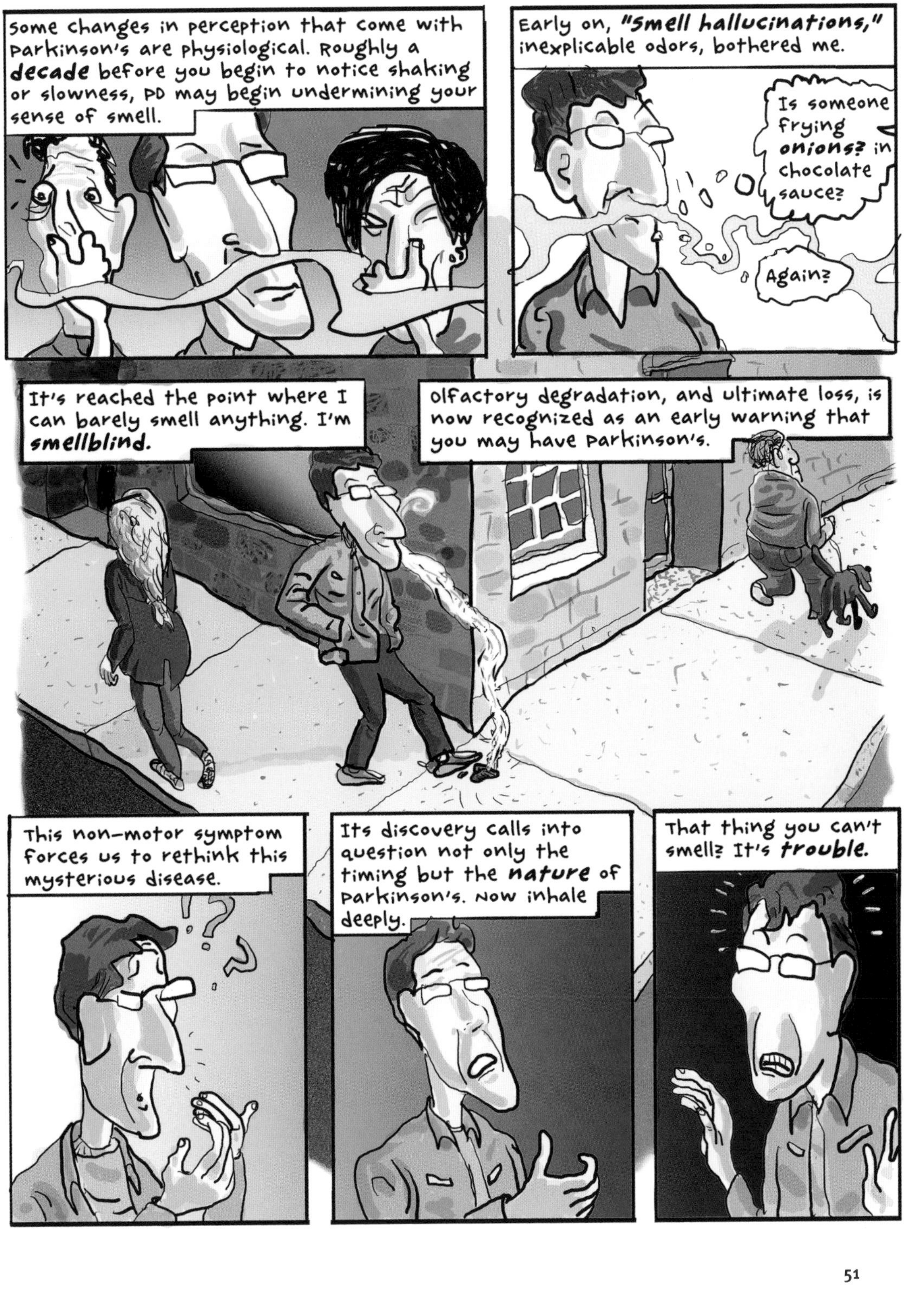
Some changes in perception that come with Parkinson's are physiological. Roughly a **decade** before you begin to notice shaking or slowness, PD may begin undermining your sense of smell.
Early on, ***"Smell hallucinations,"*** inexplicable odors, bothered me.
Is someone frying ***onions?*** in chocolate sauce?
Again?
It's reached the point where I can barely smell anything. I'm ***smellblind.***
Olfactory degradation, and ultimate loss, is now recognized as an early warning that you may have Parkinson's.
This non-motor symptom forces us to rethink this mysterious disease.
Its discovery calls into question not only the timing but the ***nature*** of Parkinson's. Now inhale deeply.
That thing you can't smell? It's ***trouble.***

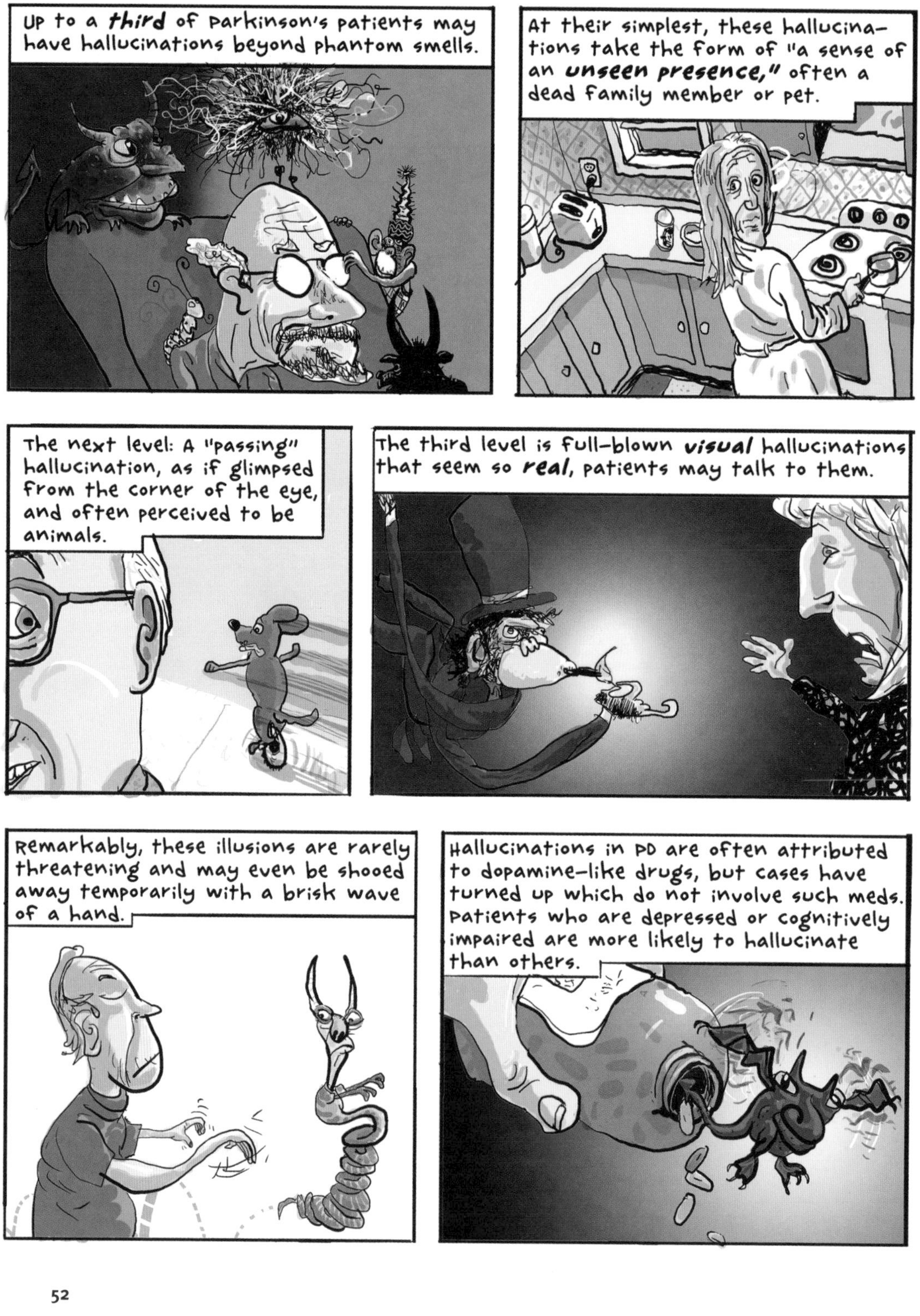
Up to a *third* of Parkinson's patients may have hallucinations beyond phantom smells.
At their simplest, these hallucinations take the form of "a sense of an *unseen presence,*" often a dead family member or pet.
The next level: A "passing" hallucination, as if glimpsed from the corner of the eye, and often perceived to be animals.
The third level is full-blown *visual* hallucinations that seem so *real*, patients may talk to them.
Remarkably, these illusions are rarely threatening and may even be shooed away temporarily with a brisk wave of a hand.
Hallucinations in PD are often attributed to dopamine-like drugs, but cases have turned up which do not involve such meds. Patients who are depressed or cognitively impaired are more likely to hallucinate than others.

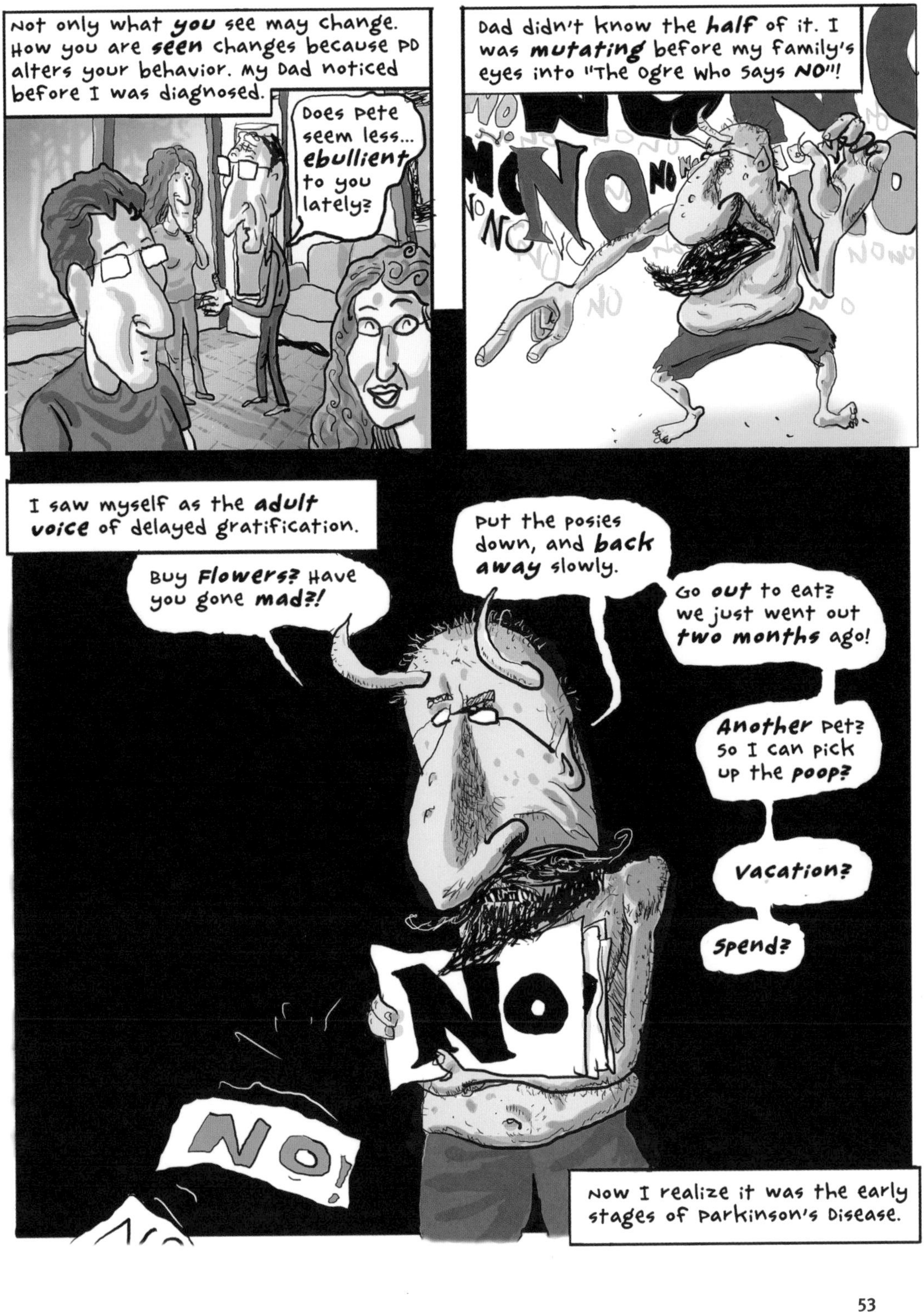
Not only what *you* see may change. How you are *seen* changes because PD alters your behavior. My Dad noticed before I was diagnosed.
Does Pete seem less... *ebullient* to you lately?
Dad didn't know the *half* of it. I was *mutating* before my family's eyes into "The Ogre Who Says *NO*"!
NO
I saw myself as the *adult voice* of delayed gratification.
Buy *Flowers?* Have you gone *mad?!*
Put the posies down, and *back away* slowly.
Go *out* to eat? we just went out *two months* ago!
Another pet? So I can pick up the *poop?*
Vacation?
Spend?
NO!
NO!
Now I realize it was the early stages of Parkinson's Disease.

The *truth* was that the ogre was slowly *smothering* those around me. An adult should find ways to say *yes*.

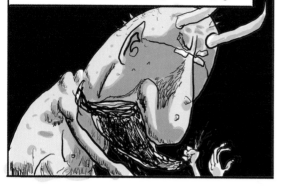

Fortunately, the ogre choked to death on his *favorite word* about the same time I got my PD meds and exercise regime together.

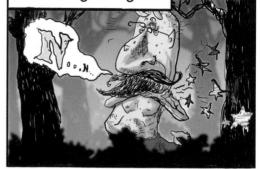

We buried him in a simple pine box.

Did you bring flowers?

Hell *no*. He'd *Hate* that!

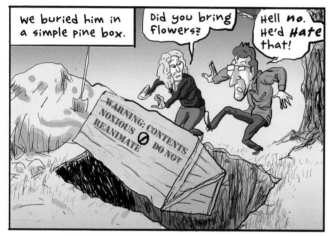

WARNING: CONTENTS NOXIOUS Ø DO NOT REANIMATE

We *do* visit his grave, to recall him, and reflect on his last words, carved plainly into his granite headstone...

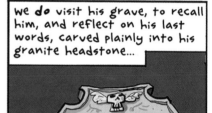

RIP
The OGRE Who says No
"CARPE DIEM"

And to make sure the bastard *stays put*.

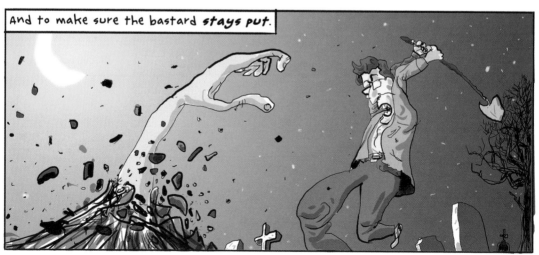

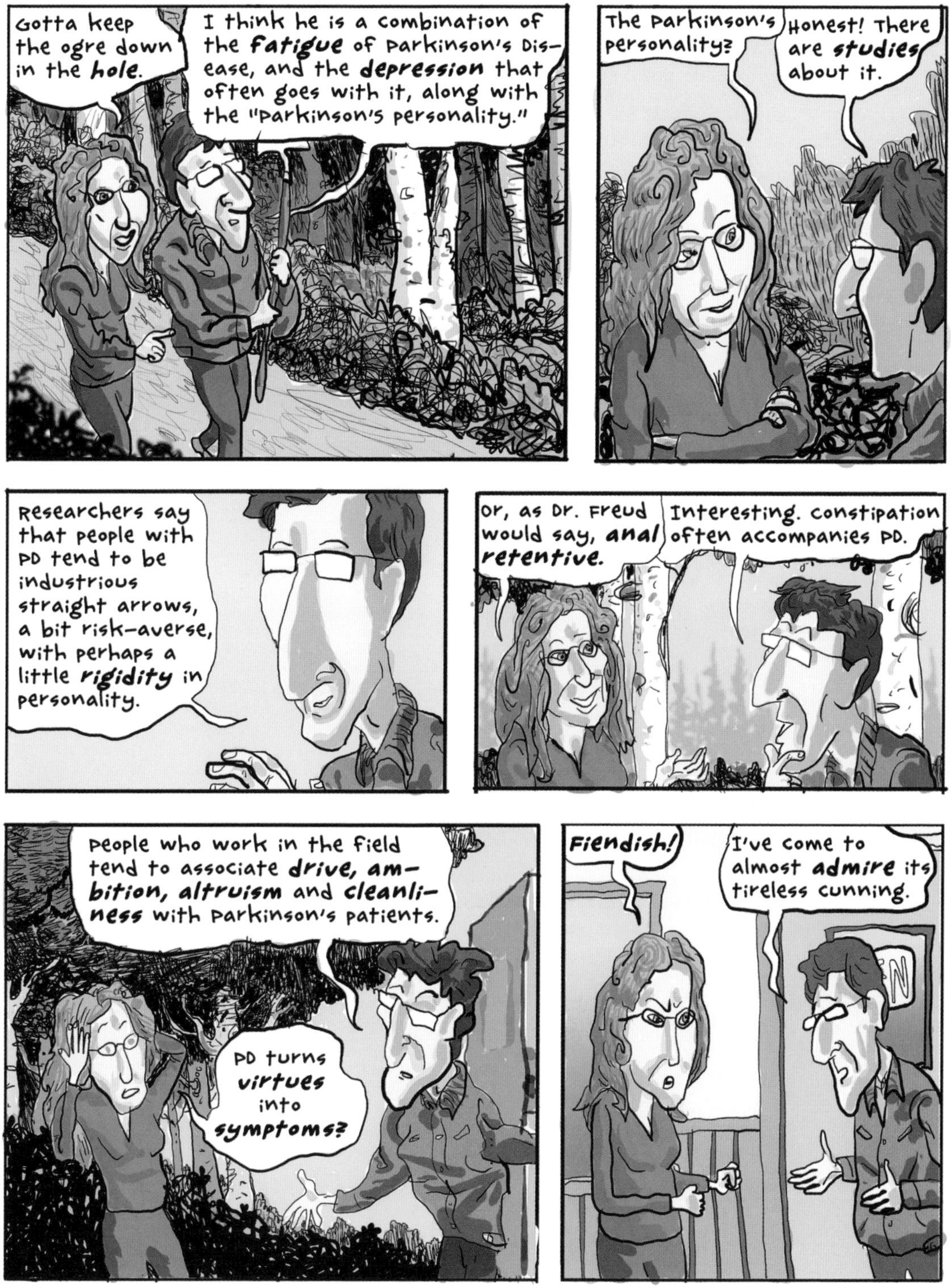
Gotta keep the ogre down in the hole.
I think he is a combination of the fatigue of Parkinson's Disease, and the depression that often goes with it, along with the "Parkinson's personality."
The Parkinson's personality?
Honest! There are studies about it.
Researchers say that people with PD tend to be industrious straight arrows, a bit risk-averse, with perhaps a little rigidity in personality.
Or, as Dr. Freud would say, anal retentive.
Interesting. Constipation often accompanies PD.
People who work in the field tend to associate drive, ambition, altruism and cleanliness with Parkinson's patients.
PD turns virtues into symptoms?
Fiendish!
I've come to almost admire its tireless cunning.

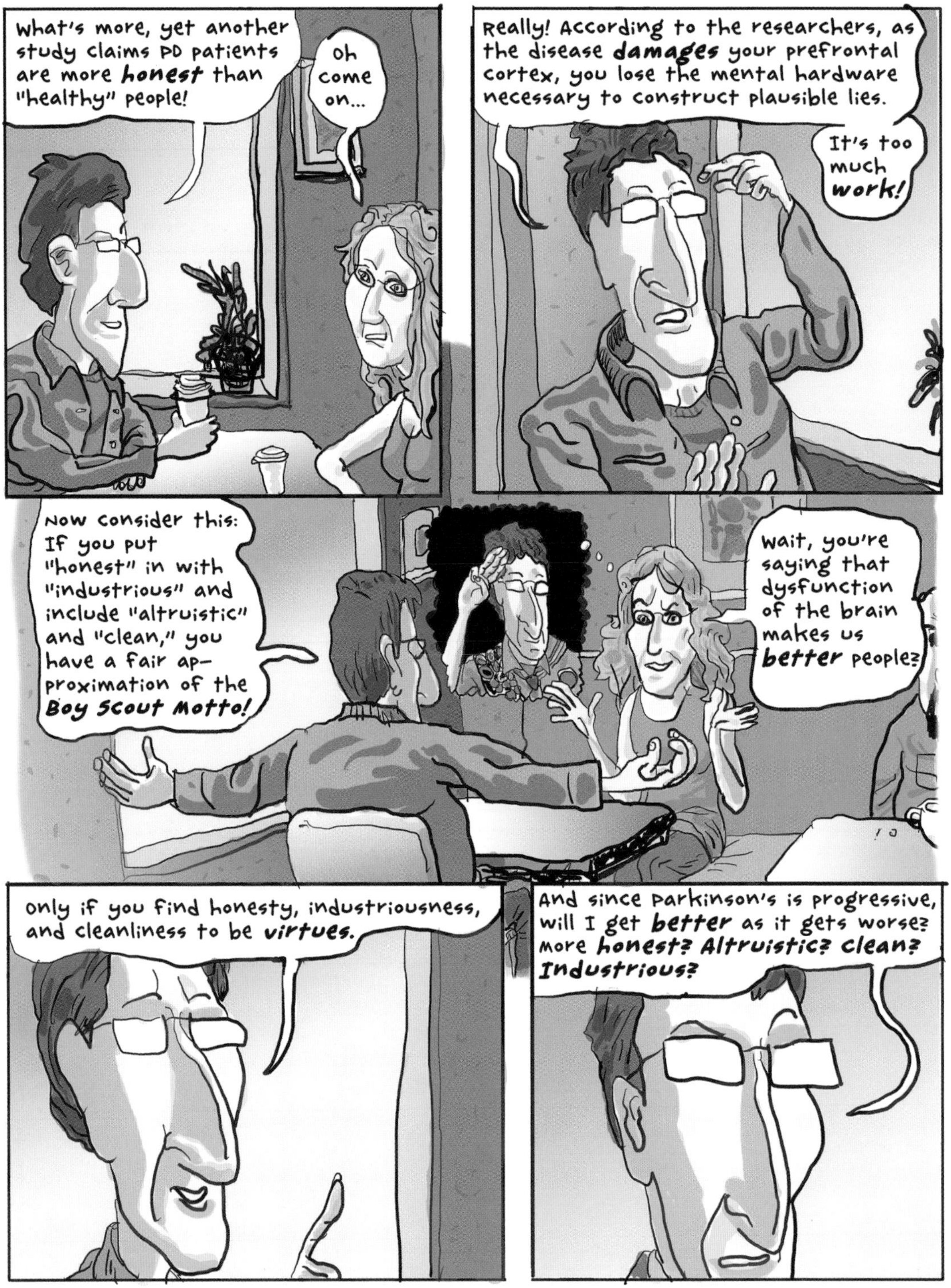
What's more, yet another study claims PD patients are more honest than "healthy" people!
Oh come on...
Really! According to the researchers, as the disease damages your prefrontal cortex, you lose the mental hardware necessary to construct plausible lies.
It's too much work!
Now consider this: If you put "honest" in with "industrious" and include "altruistic" and "clean," you have a fair approximation of the Boy Scout Motto!
Wait, you're saying that dysfunction of the brain makes us better people?
Only if you find honesty, industriousness, and cleanliness to be virtues.
And since Parkinson's is progressive, will I get better as it gets worse? More honest? Altruistic? Clean? Industrious?

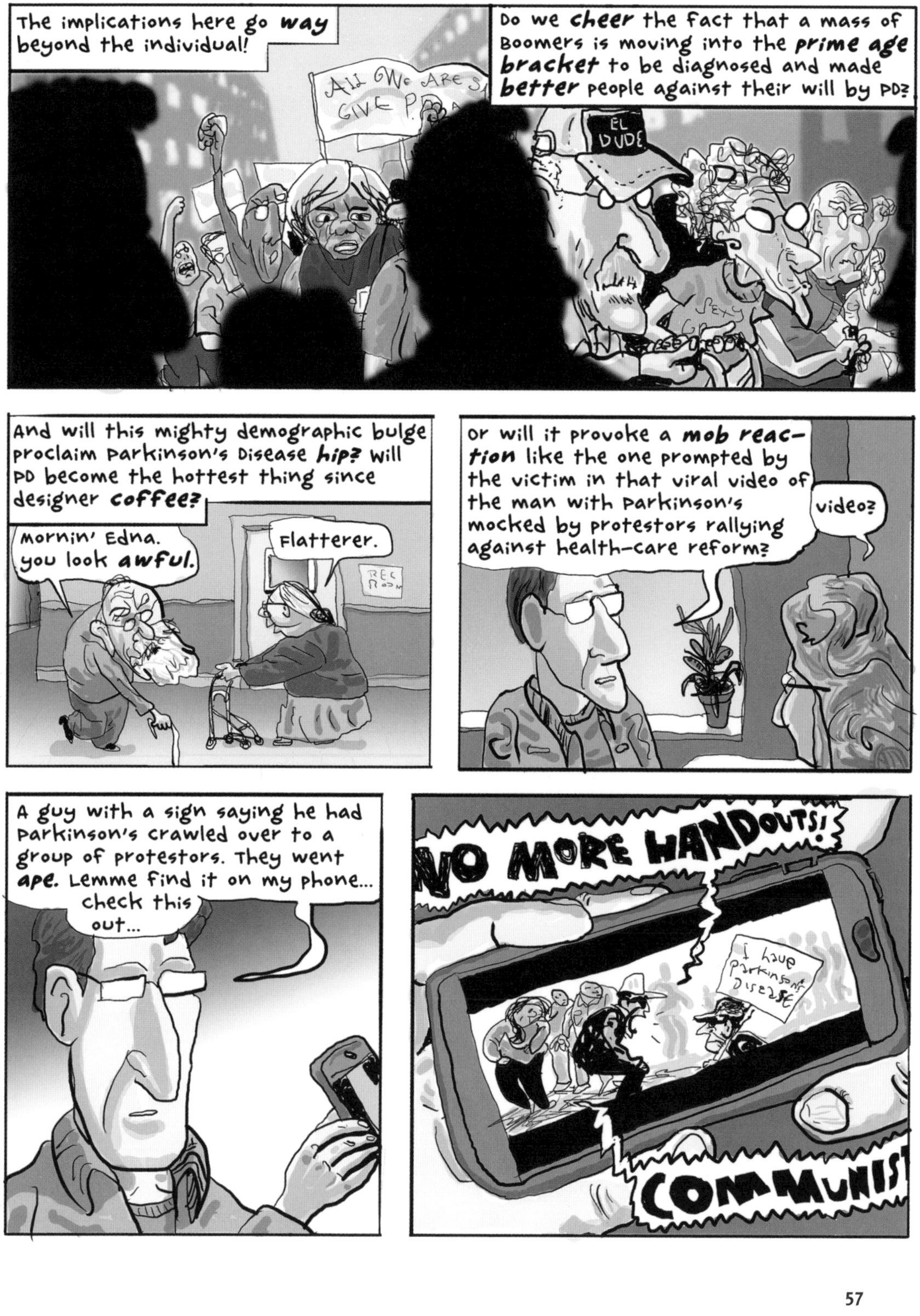
The implications here go way beyond the individual!
Do we cheer the fact that a mass of Boomers is moving into the prime age bracket to be diagnosed and made better people against their will by PD?
EL DUDE
And will this mighty demographic bulge proclaim Parkinson's Disease hip? Will PD become the hottest thing since designer coffee?
Mornin' Edna. You look awful.
Flatterer.
Or will it provoke a mob reaction like the one prompted by the victim in that viral video of the man with Parkinson's mocked by protestors rallying against health-care reform?
Video?
A guy with a sign saying he had Parkinson's crawled over to a group of protestors. They went ape. Lemme find it on my phone... check this out...
NO MORE HANDOUTS!
I have Parkinson's Disease
COMMUNIST

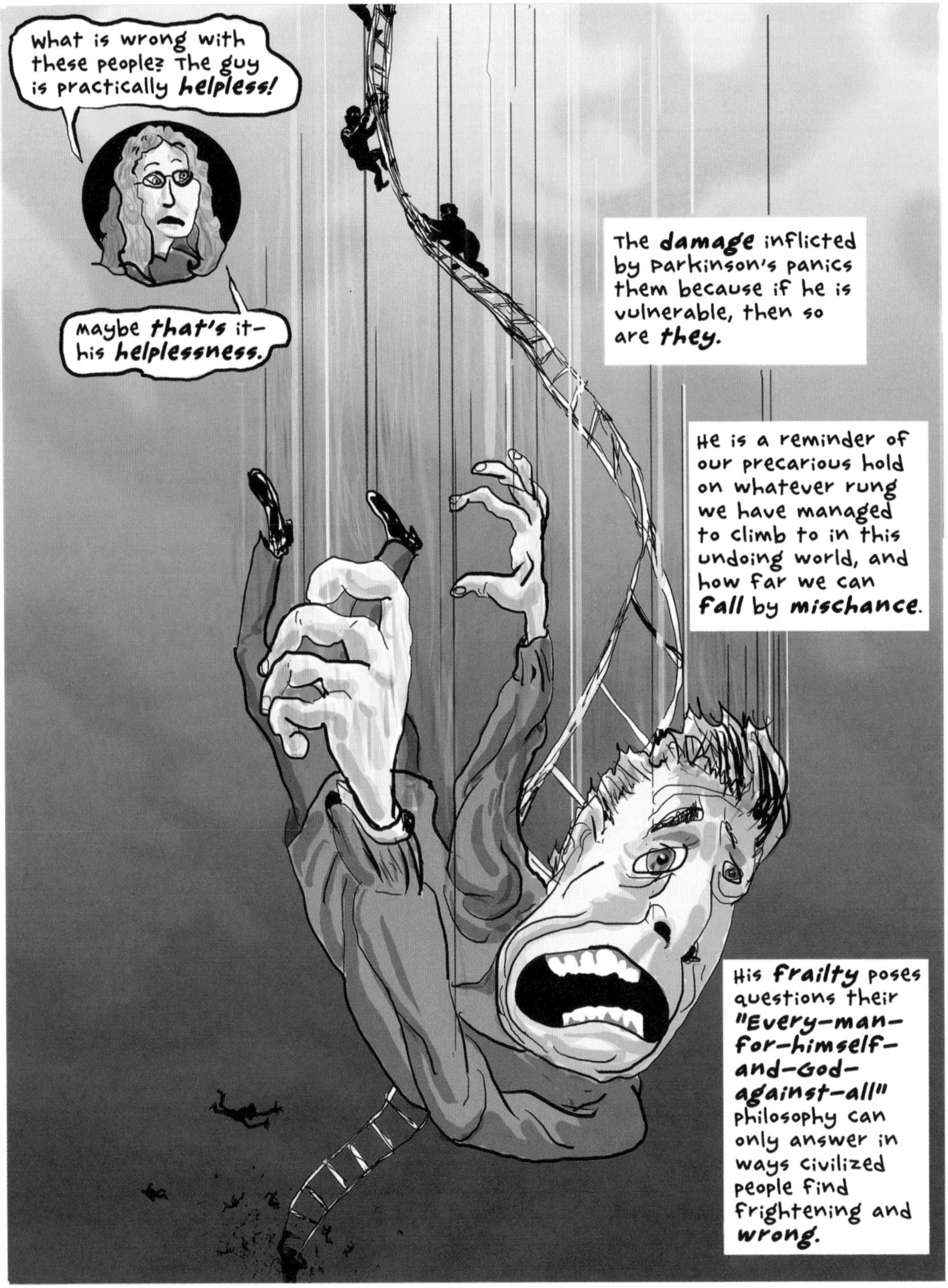
What is wrong with these people? The guy is practically helpless!
Maybe that's it—his helplessness.
The damage inflicted by Parkinson's panics them because if he is vulnerable, then so are they.
He is a reminder of our precarious hold on whatever rung we have managed to climb to in this undoing world, and how far we can fall by mischance.
His frailty poses questions their "Every-man-for-himself-and-God-against-all" philosophy can only answer in ways civilized people find frightening and wrong.

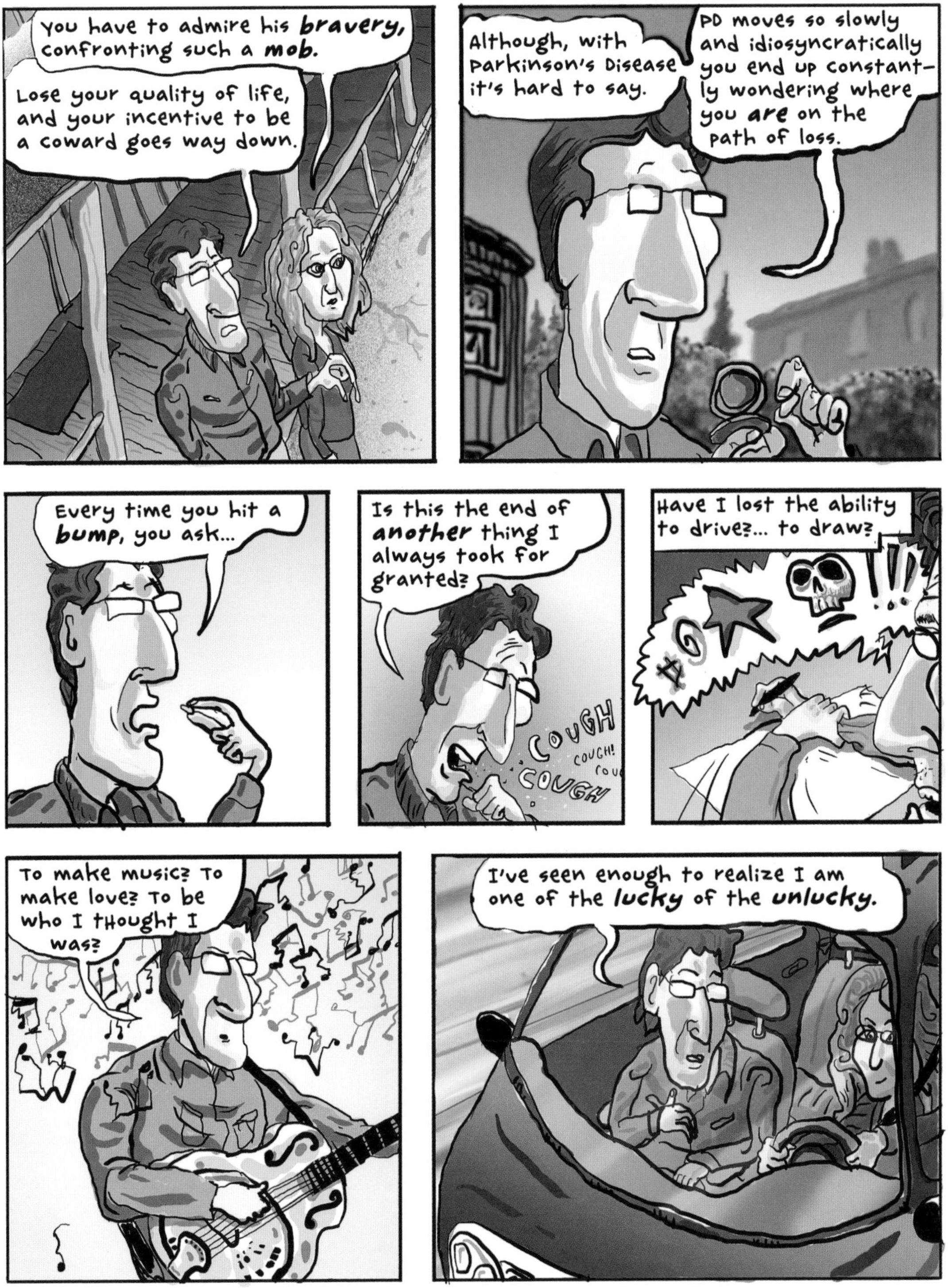
You have to admire his bravery, confronting such a mob.
Lose your quality of life, and your incentive to be a coward goes way down.
Although, with Parkinson's Disease it's hard to say.
PD moves so slowly and idiosyncratically you end up constantly wondering where you are on the path of loss.
Every time you hit a bump, you ask...
Is this the end of another thing I always took for granted?
COUGH
COUGH!
COUGH
Have I lost the ability to drive?... to draw?
To make music? To make love? To be who I thought I was?
I've seen enough to realize I am one of the lucky of the unlucky.

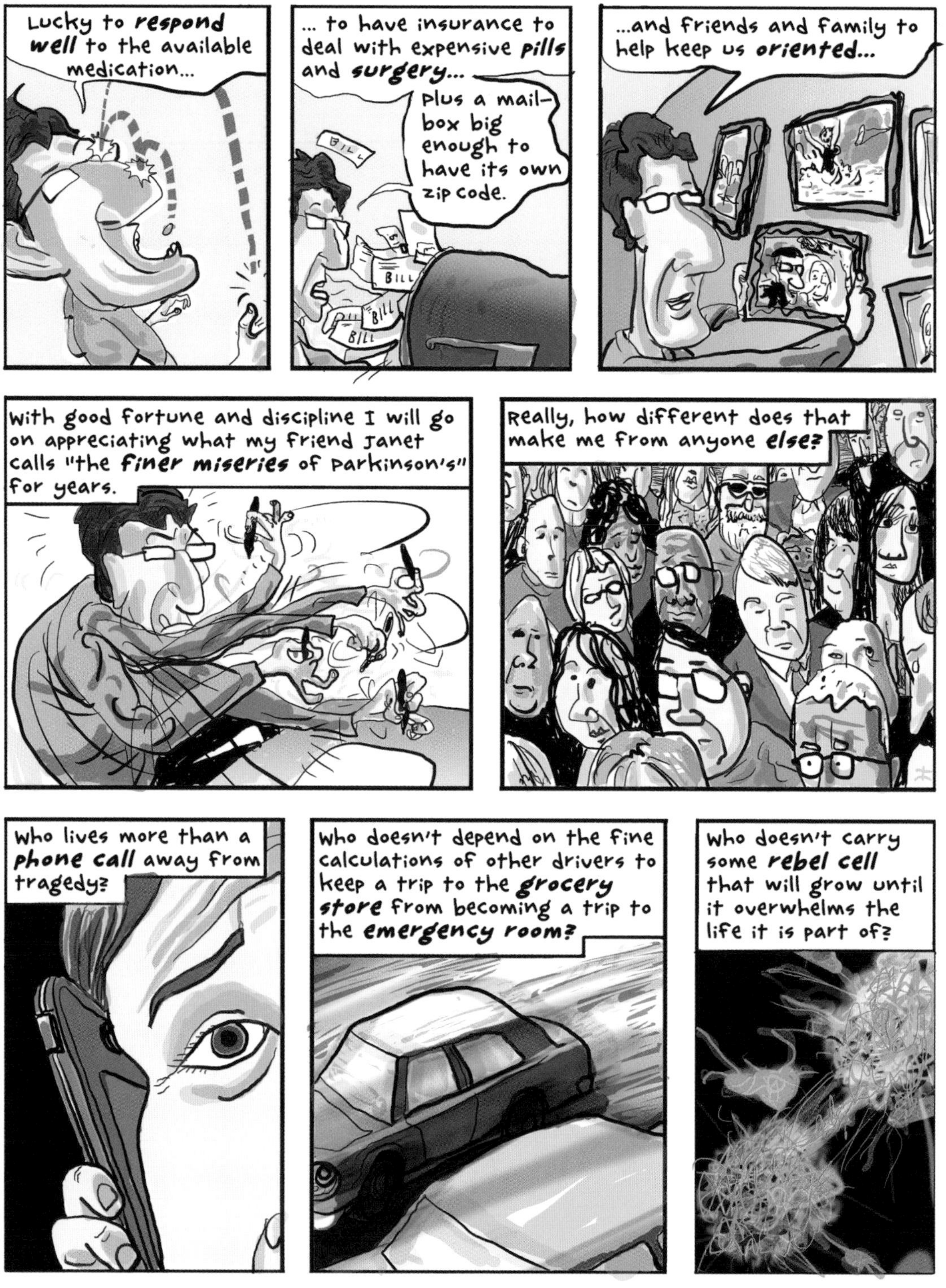
Lucky to respond well to the available medication...
... to have insurance to deal with expensive pills and surgery...
Plus a mail-box big enough to have its own zip code.
BILL
BILL
BILL
BILL
...and friends and family to help keep us oriented...
With good fortune and discipline I will go on appreciating what my friend Janet calls "the finer miseries of Parkinson's" for years.
Really, how different does that make me from anyone else?
Who lives more than a phone call away from tragedy?
Who doesn't depend on the fine calculations of other drivers to keep a trip to the grocery store from becoming a trip to the emergency room?
Who doesn't carry some rebel cell that will grow until it overwhelms the life it is part of?

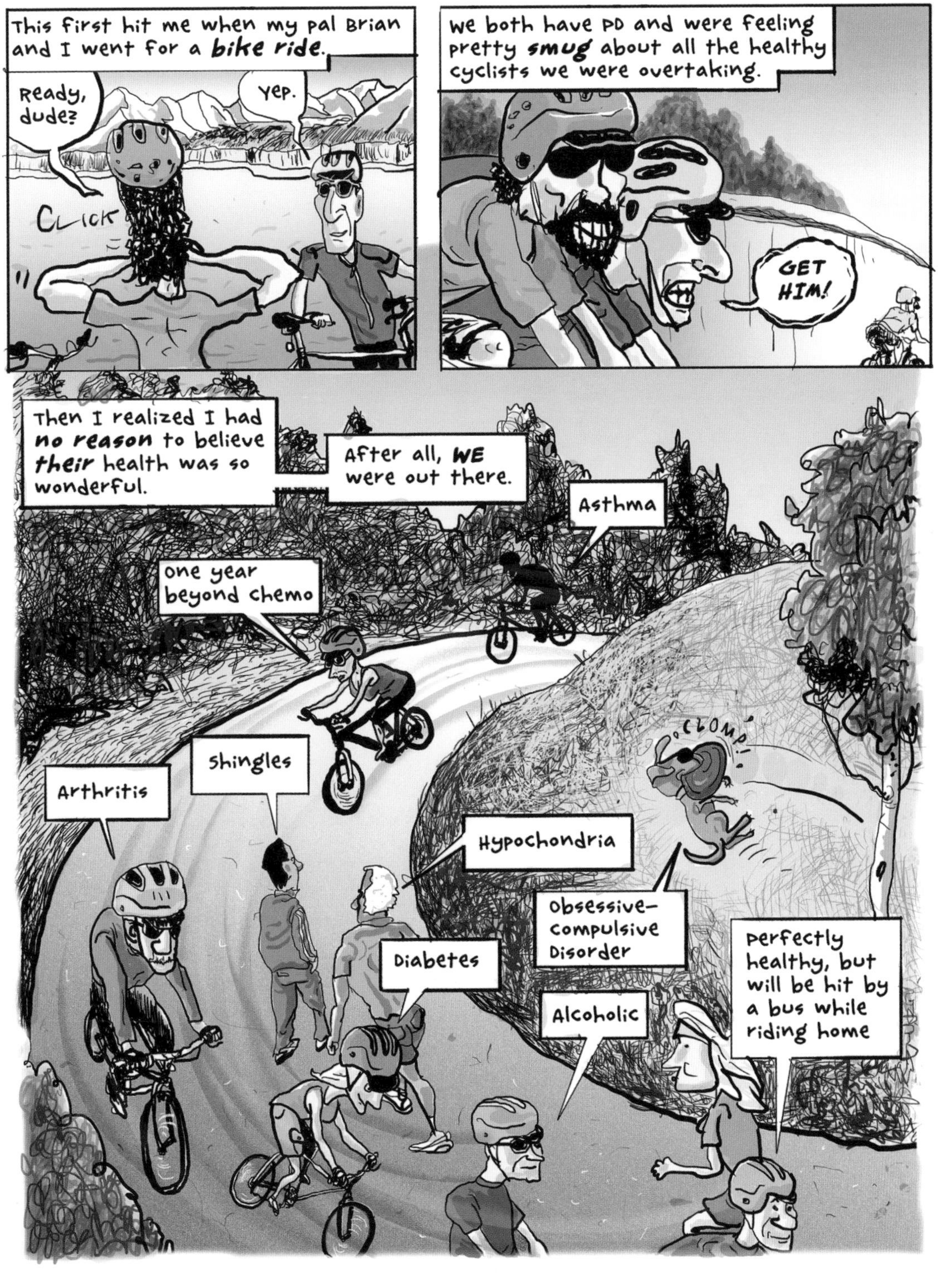
This first hit me when my pal Brian and I went for a **bike ride**.
Ready, dude?
Yep.
CLICK
We both have PD and were feeling pretty **smug** about all the healthy cyclists we were overtaking.
GET HIM!
Then I realized I had **no reason** to believe **their** health was so wonderful.
After all, **WE** were out there.
Asthma
one year beyond chemo
CLOMP!
Shingles
Arthritis
Hypochondria
Obsessive-compulsive Disorder
Diabetes
Perfectly healthy, but will be hit by a bus while riding home
Alcoholic

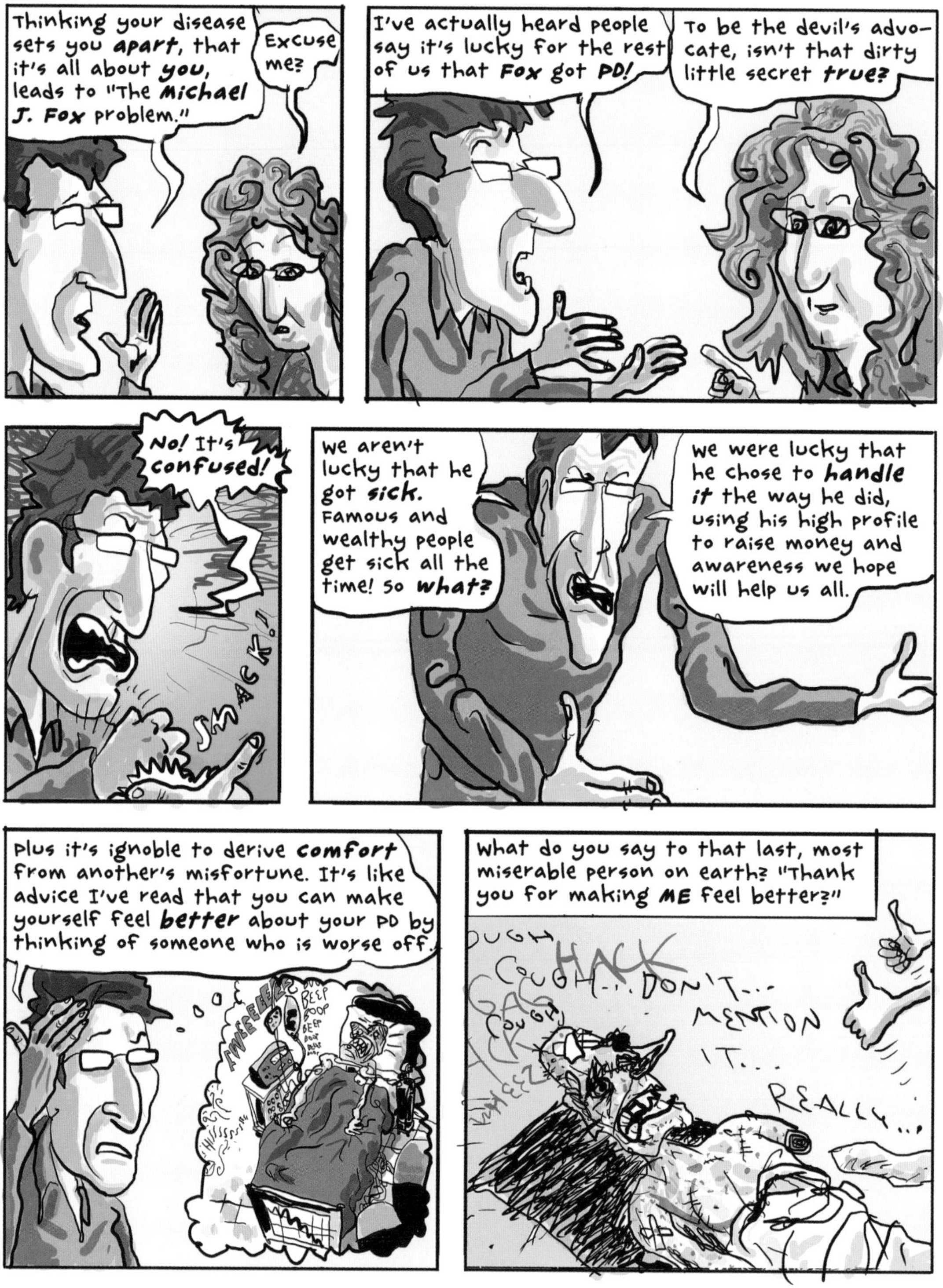
Thinking your disease sets you apart, that it's all about you, leads to "The Michael J. Fox problem."
Excuse me?
I've actually heard people say it's lucky for the rest of us that Fox got PD!
To be the devil's advocate, isn't that dirty little secret true?
No! It's confused!
SMACK!
We aren't lucky that he got sick. Famous and wealthy people get sick all the time! So what?
We were lucky that he chose to handle it the way he did, using his high profile to raise money and awareness we hope will help us all.
Plus it's ignoble to derive comfort from another's misfortune. It's like advice I've read that you can make yourself feel better about your PD by thinking of someone who is worse off.
BEEP BOOP
What do you say to that last, most miserable person on earth? "Thank you for making ME feel better?"
HACK
COUGH... DON'T... MENTION IT... REALLY...

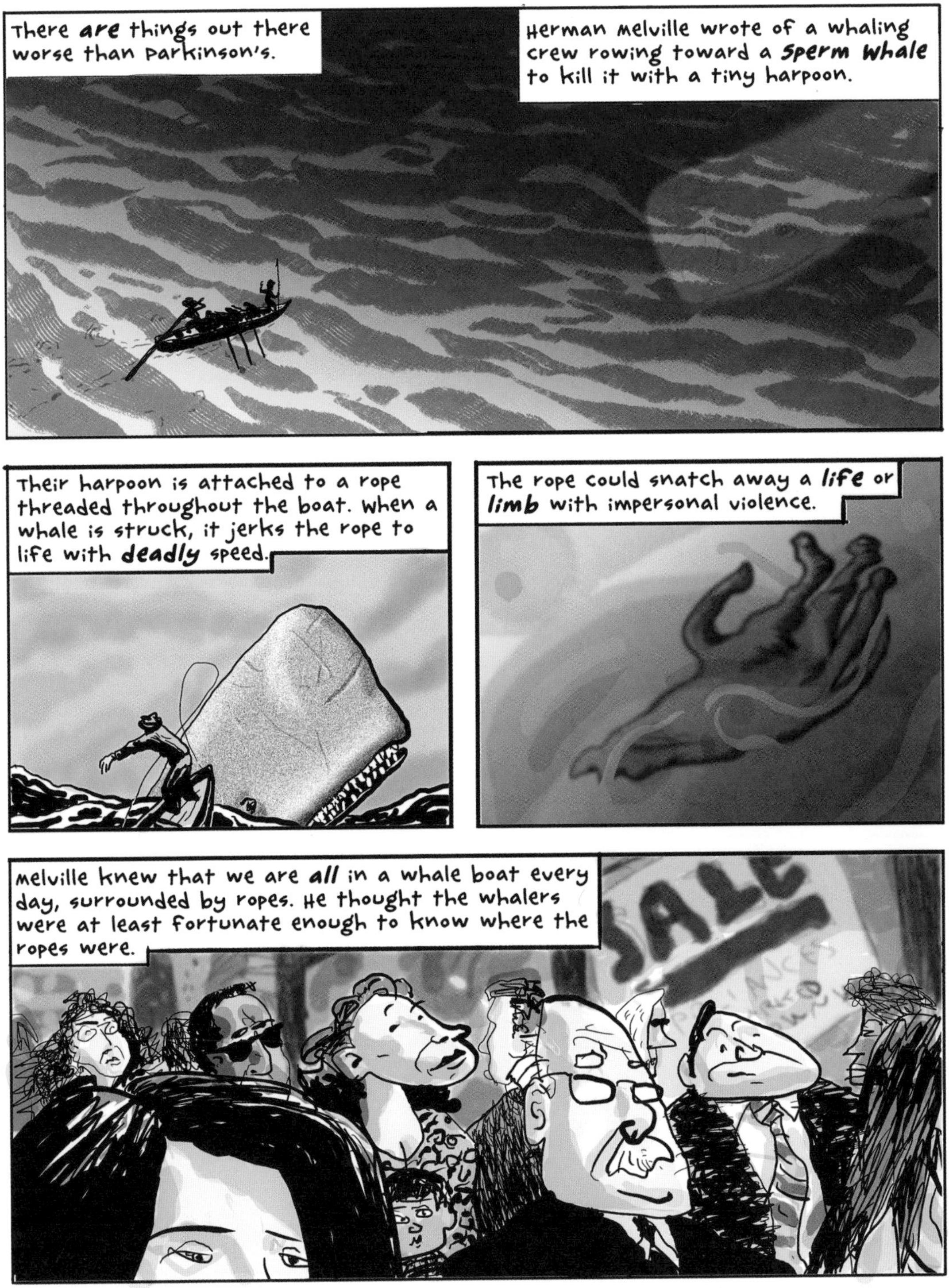
There **are** things out there worse than Parkinson's.
Herman Melville wrote of a whaling crew rowing toward a **sperm whale** to kill it with a tiny harpoon.
Their harpoon is attached to a rope threaded throughout the boat. When a whale is struck, it jerks the rope to life with **deadly** speed.
The rope could snatch away a **life** or **limb** with impersonal violence.
Melville knew that we are **all** in a whale boat every day, surrounded by ropes. He thought the whalers were at least fortunate enough to know where the ropes were.

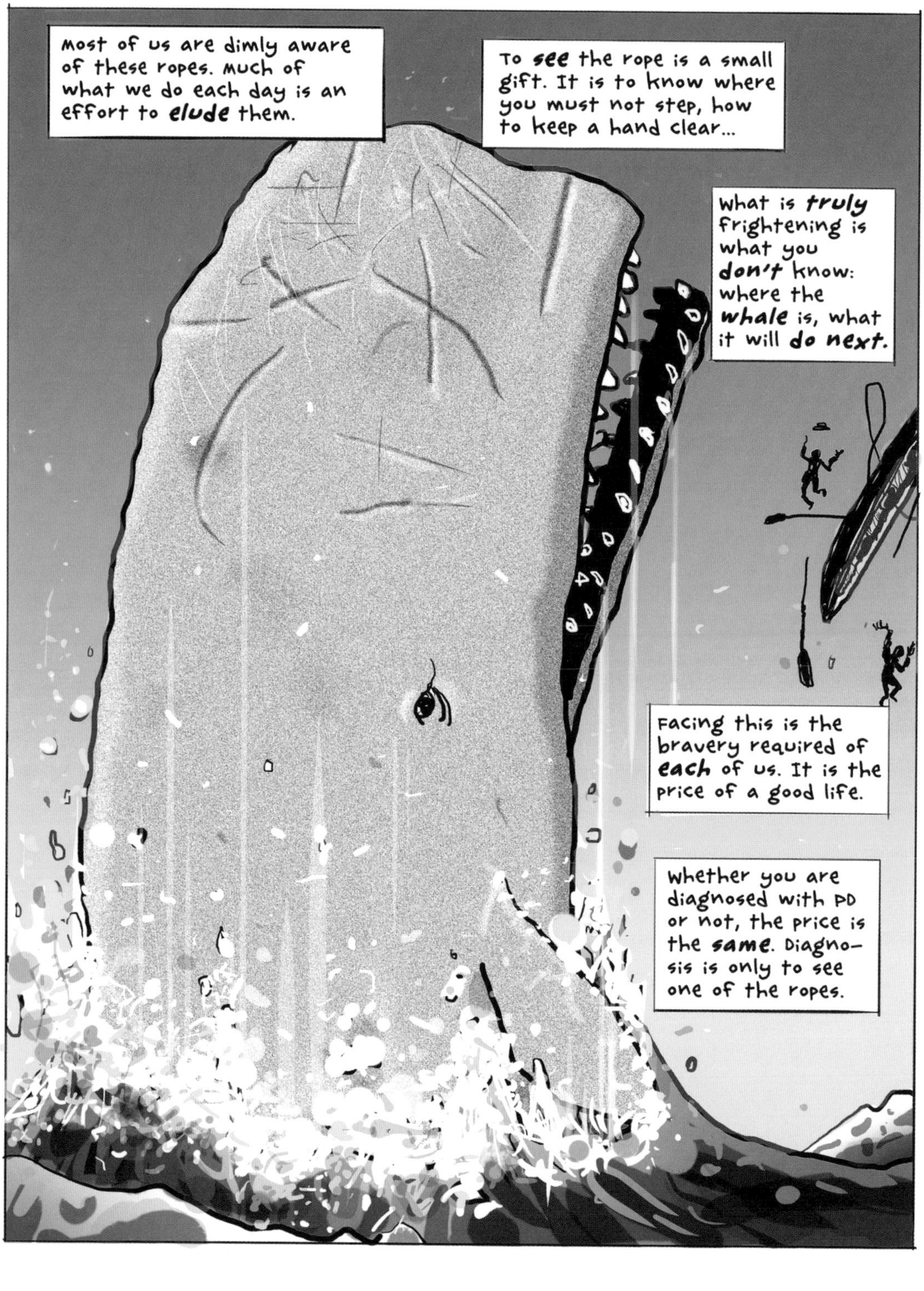
most of us are dimly aware of these ropes. much of what we do each day is an effort to elude them.
To see the rope is a small gift. It is to know where you must not step, how to keep a hand clear...
what is truly frightening is what you don't know: where the whale is, what it will do next.
Facing this is the bravery required of each of us. It is the price of a good life.
whether you are diagnosed with PD or not, the price is the same. Diagnosis is only to see one of the ropes.

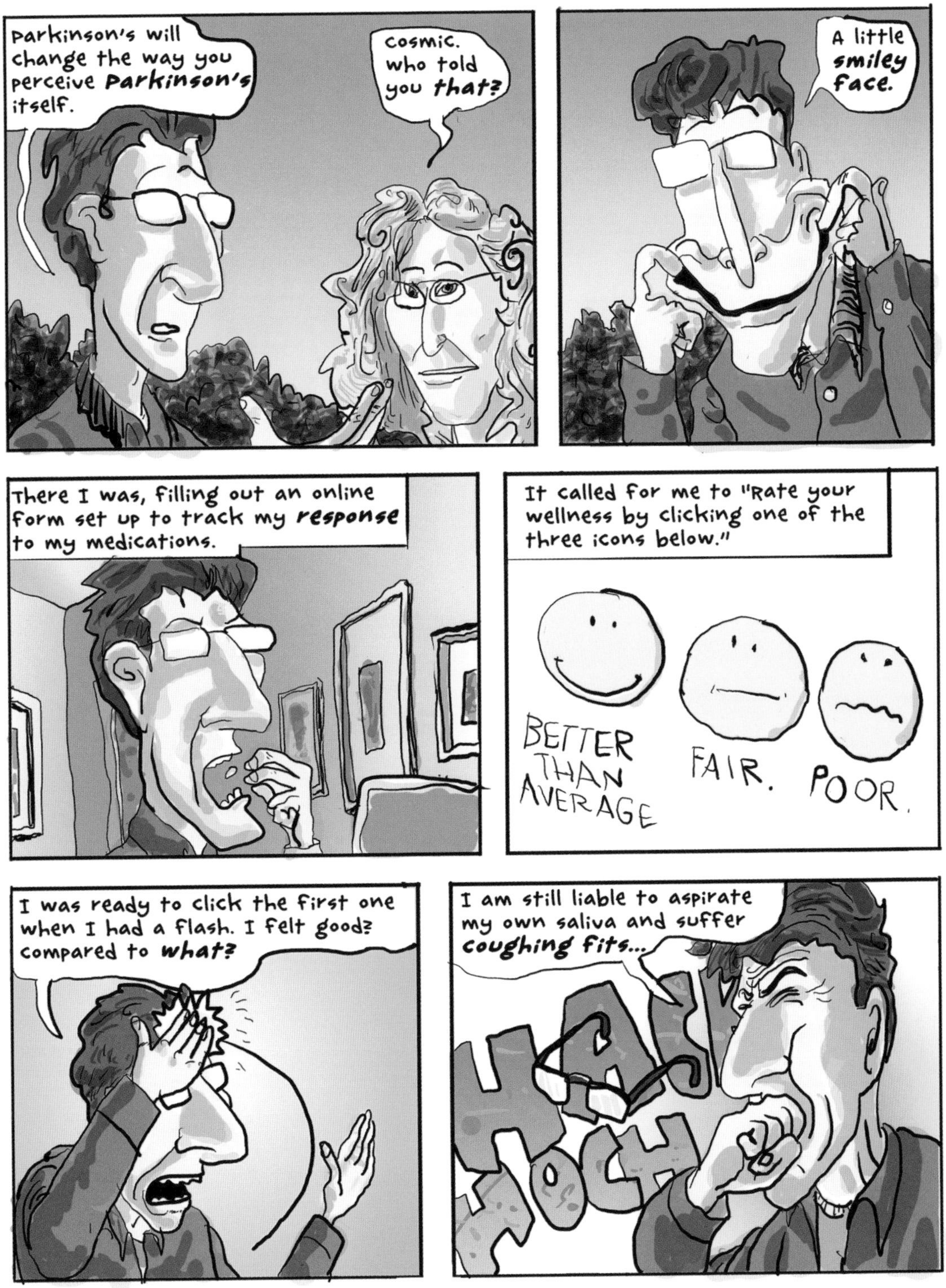
Parkinson's will change the way you perceive Parkinson's itself.
Cosmic. Who told you that?
A little smiley face.
There I was, filling out an online form set up to track my response to my medications.
It called for me to "Rate your wellness by clicking one of the three icons below."
BETTER THAN AVERAGE
FAIR.
POOR.
I was ready to click the first one when I had a flash. I felt good? Compared to what?
I am still liable to aspirate my own saliva and suffer coughing fits...

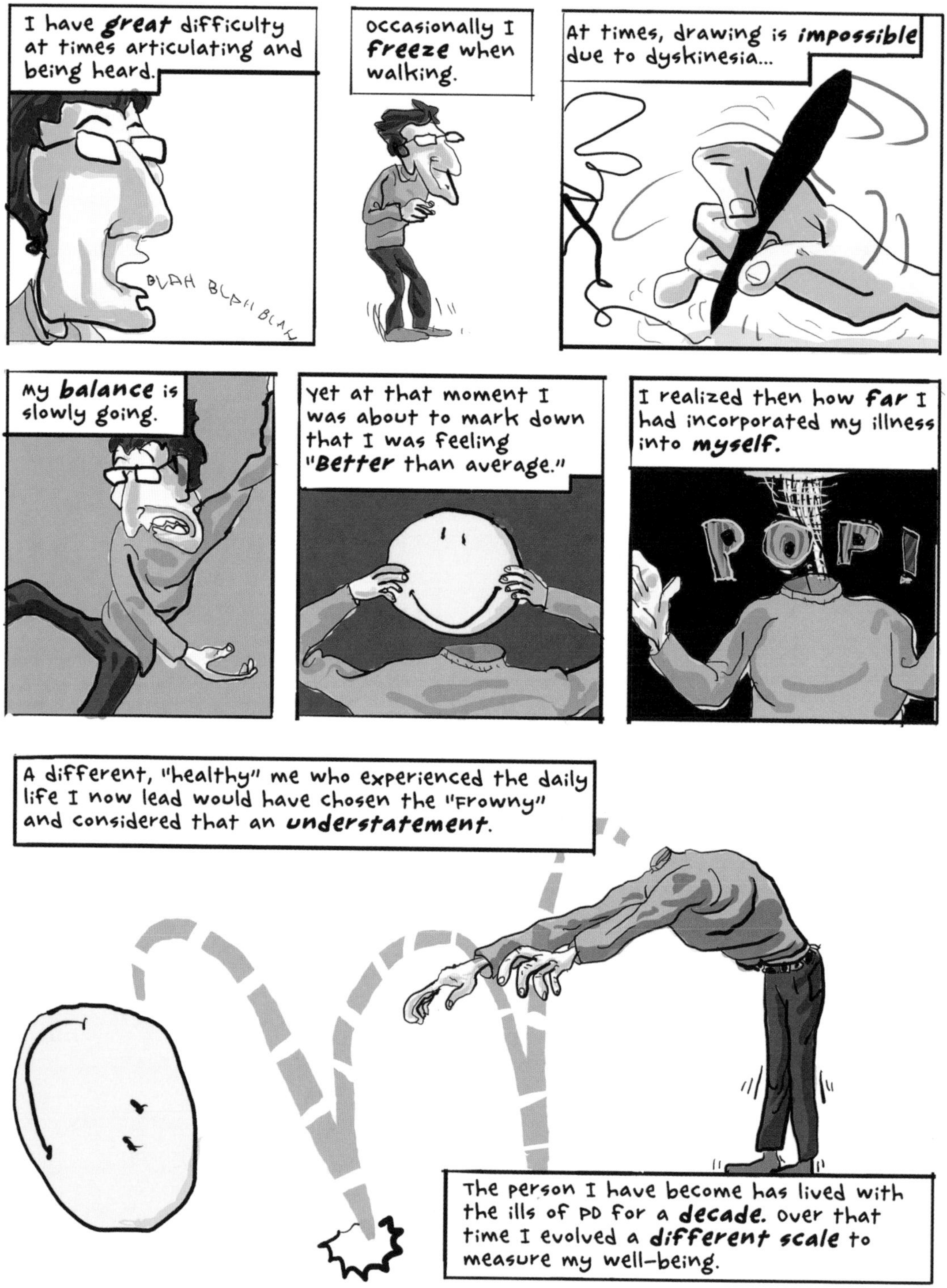
I have great difficulty at times articulating and being heard.
BLAH BLAH BLAH
Occasionally I freeze when walking.
At times, drawing is impossible due to dyskinesia...
My balance is slowly going.
Yet at that moment I was about to mark down that I was feeling "Better than average."
I realized then how far I had incorporated my illness into myself.
POP!
A different, "healthy" me who experienced the daily life I now lead would have chosen the "Frowny" and considered that an understatement.
The person I have become has lived with the ills of PD for a decade. Over that time I evolved a different scale to measure my well-being.

Humans are **adapters**. We can live in Arctic ice, or the jungles of the tropics. Where adaptation calls for it, we will even live as nomads, ***without*** a home.

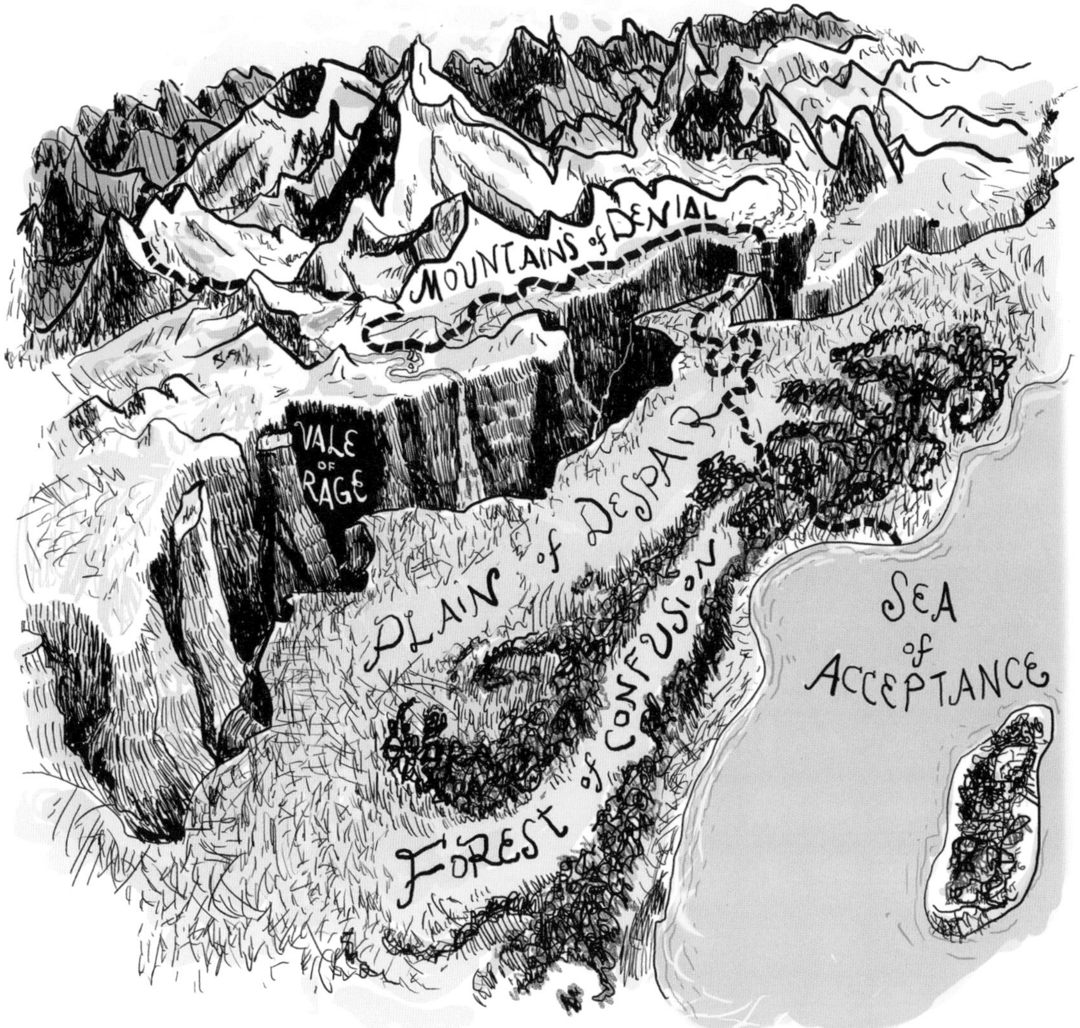
MOUNTAINS of DENIAL
VALE of RAGE
PLAIN of DESPAIR
FOREST of CONFUSION
SEA of ACCEPTANCE

Thoreau wrote, "I have travelled a good deal in Concord." I've come further than I thought possible in adapting to Parkinson's Disease. How far? All the way to a place I'd lost the capacity to even imagine.

6. Island of the Caring and Competent

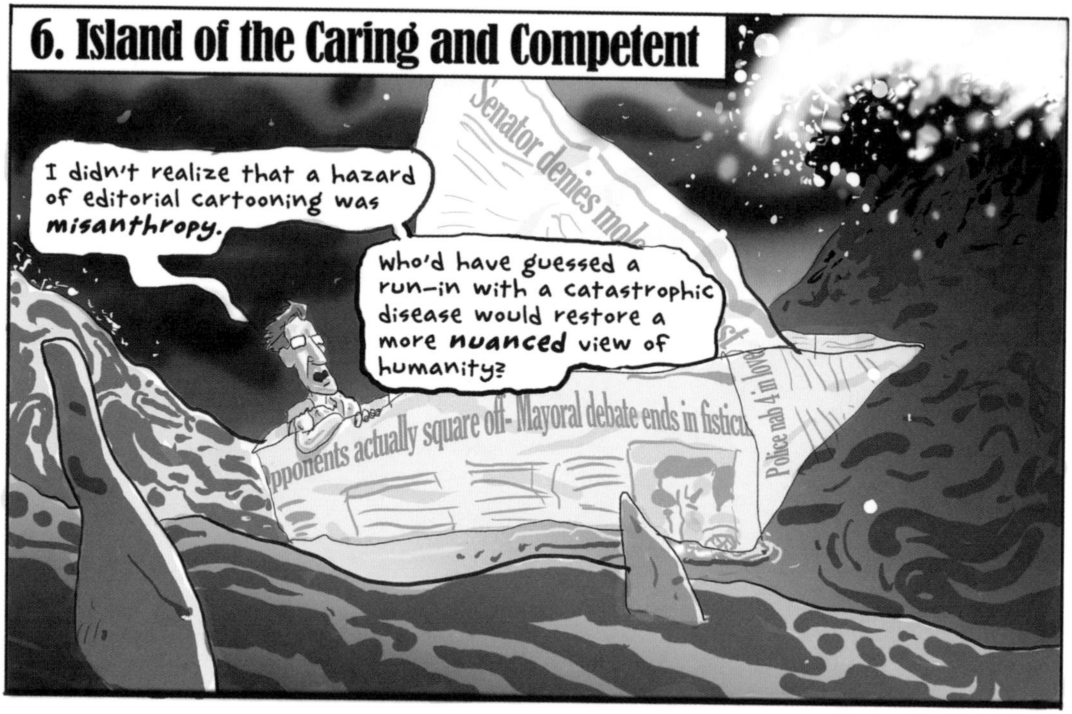

Senator denies mole
I didn't realize that a hazard of editorial cartooning was misanthropy.
Who'd have guessed a run-in with a catastrophic disease would restore a more nuanced view of humanity?
Opponents actually square off- Mayoral debate ends in fisticu
Police nab 4 in love

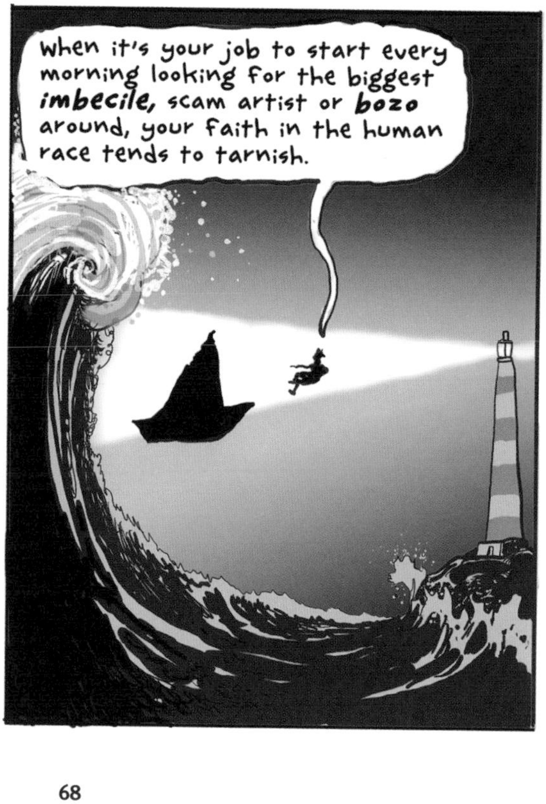

When it's your job to start every morning looking for the biggest imbecile, scam artist or bozo around, your faith in the human race tends to tarnish.

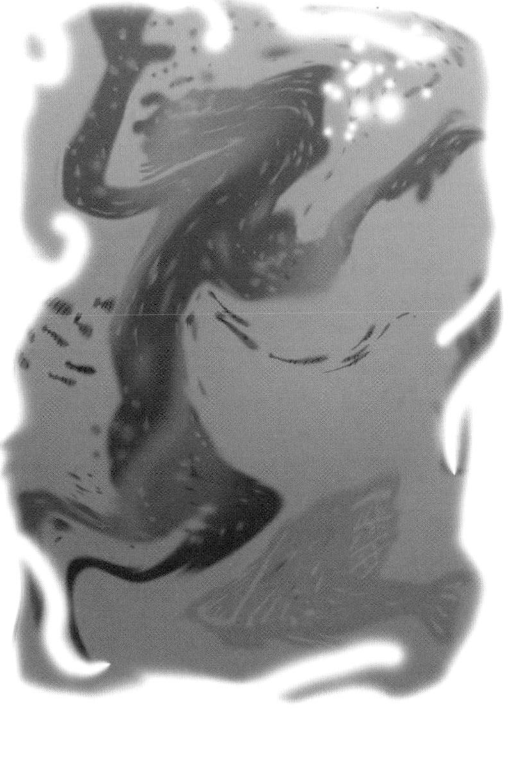

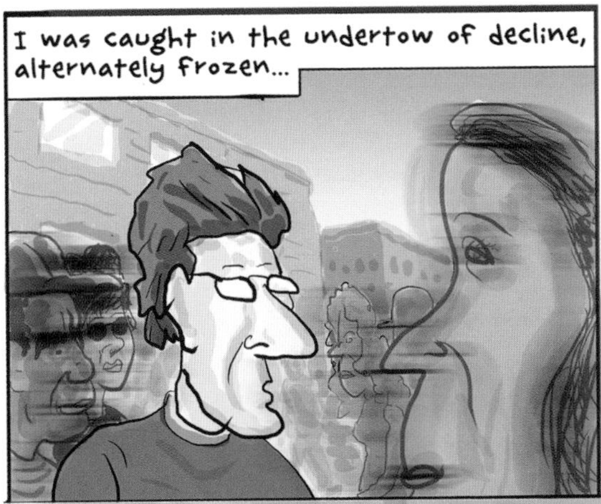
I was caught in the undertow of decline, alternately frozen...

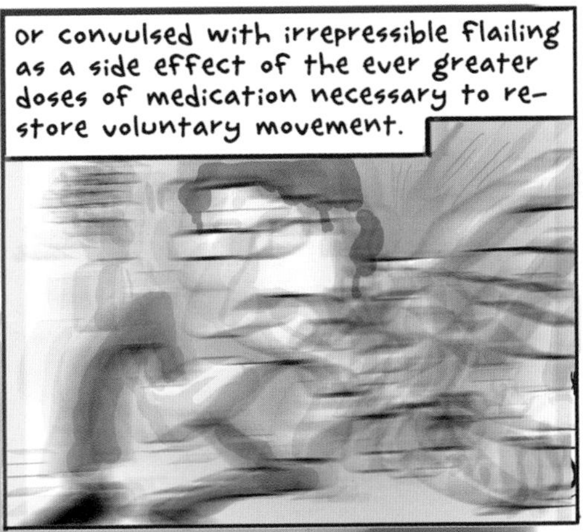
or convulsed with irrepressible flailing as a side effect of the ever greater doses of medication necessary to restore voluntary movement.

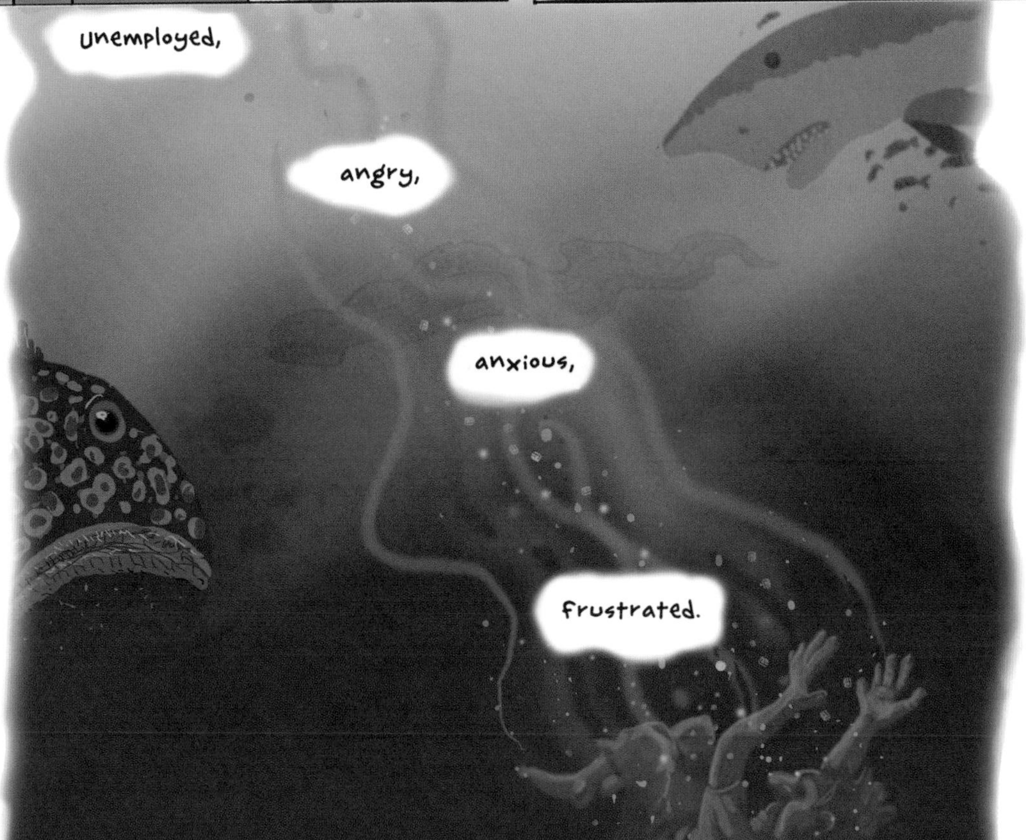
unemployed,
angry,
anxious,
frustrated.

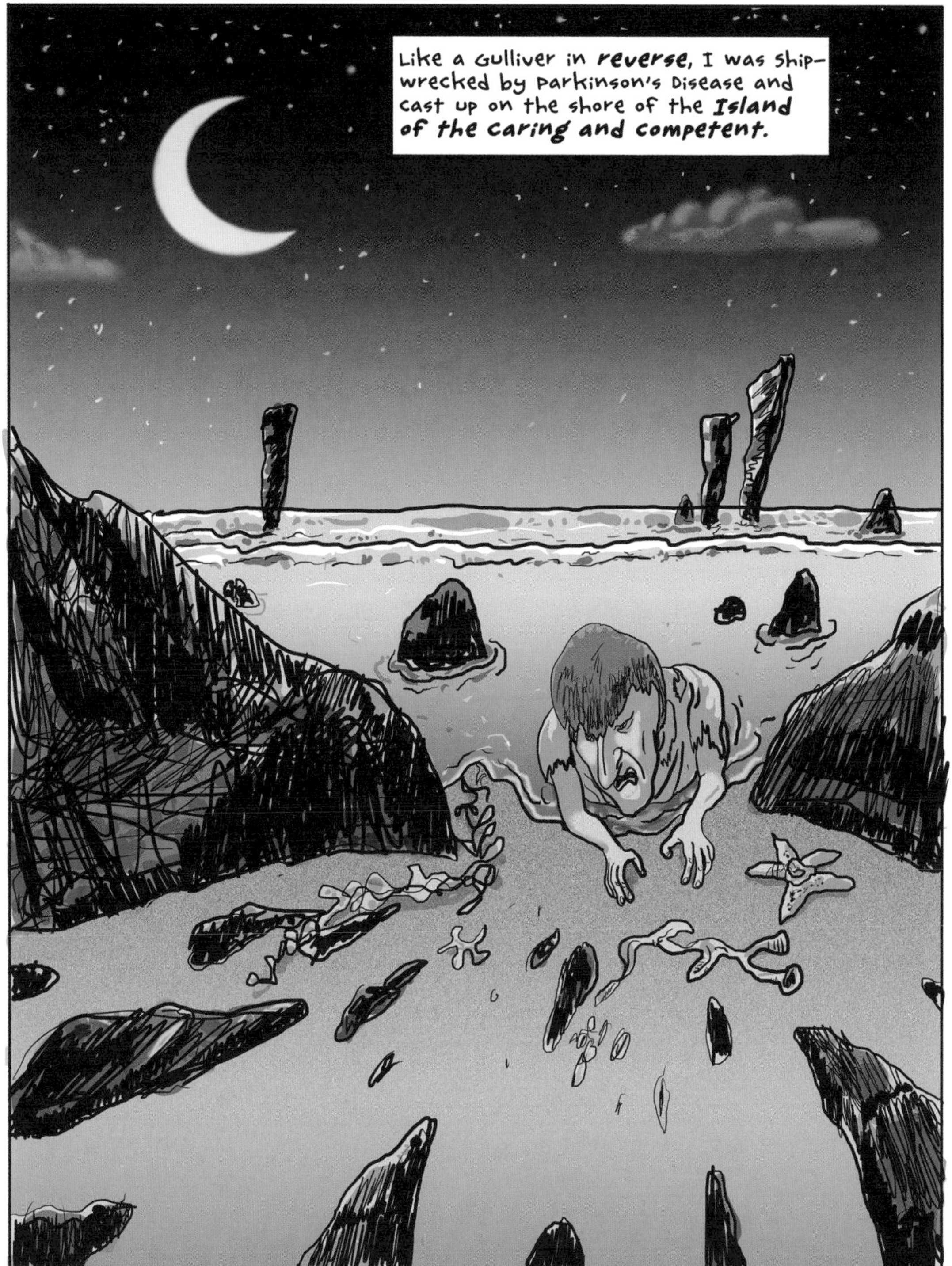
Like a Gulliver in *reverse*, I was ship-wrecked by Parkinson's Disease and cast up on the shore of the ***Island of the caring and competent.***

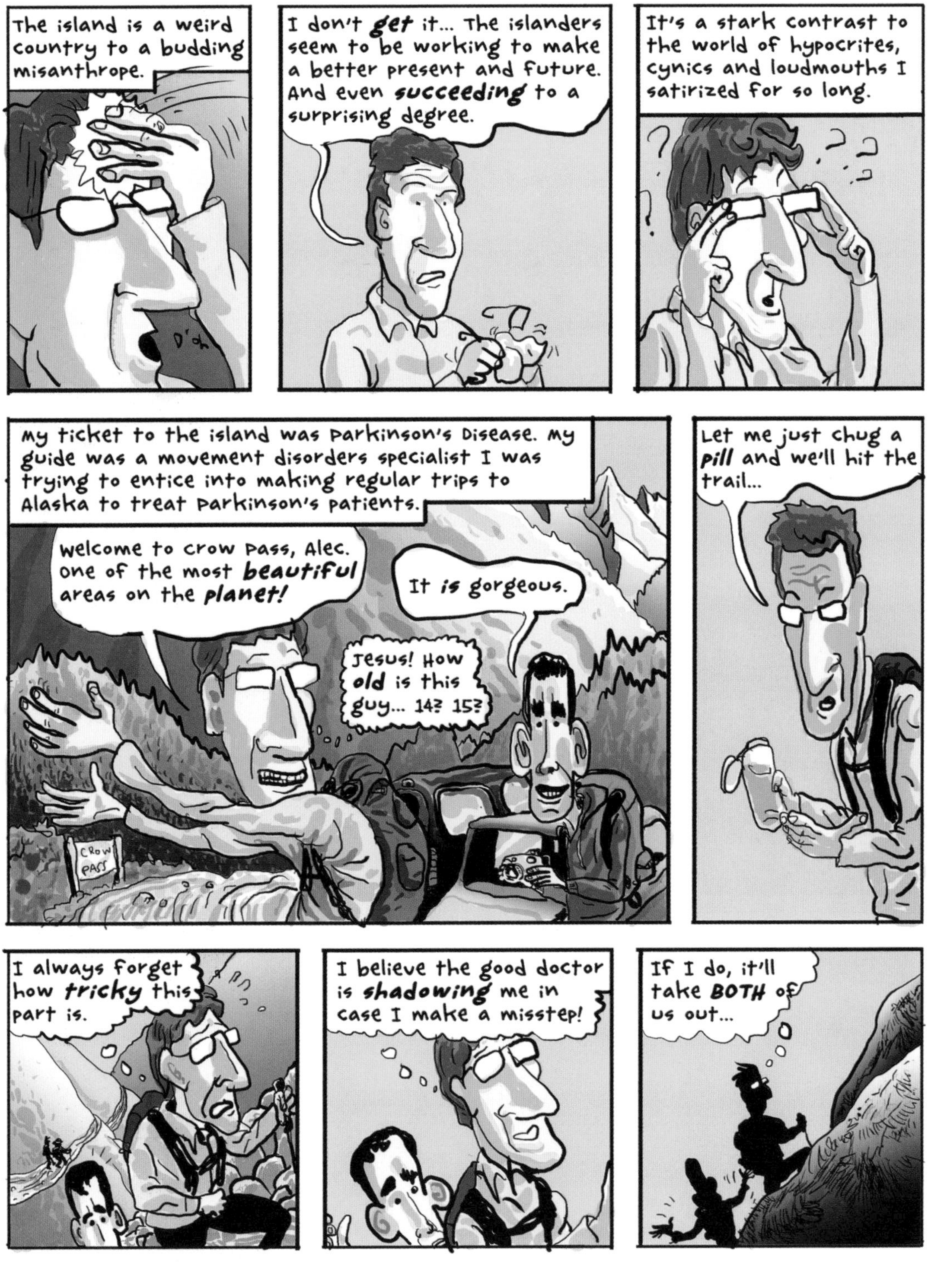
The island is a weird country to a budding misanthrope.
D'oh
I don't get it... The islanders seem to be working to make a better present and future. And even succeeding to a surprising degree.
It's a stark contrast to the world of hypocrites, cynics and loudmouths I satirized for so long.
My ticket to the island was Parkinson's Disease. My guide was a movement disorders specialist I was trying to entice into making regular trips to Alaska to treat Parkinson's patients.
Welcome to Crow Pass, Alec. One of the most beautiful areas on the planet!
It is gorgeous.
Jesus! How old is this guy... 14? 15?
CROW PASS
Let me just chug a pill and we'll hit the trail...
I always forget how tricky this part is.
I believe the good doctor is shadowing me in case I make a misstep!
If I do, it'll take BOTH of us out...

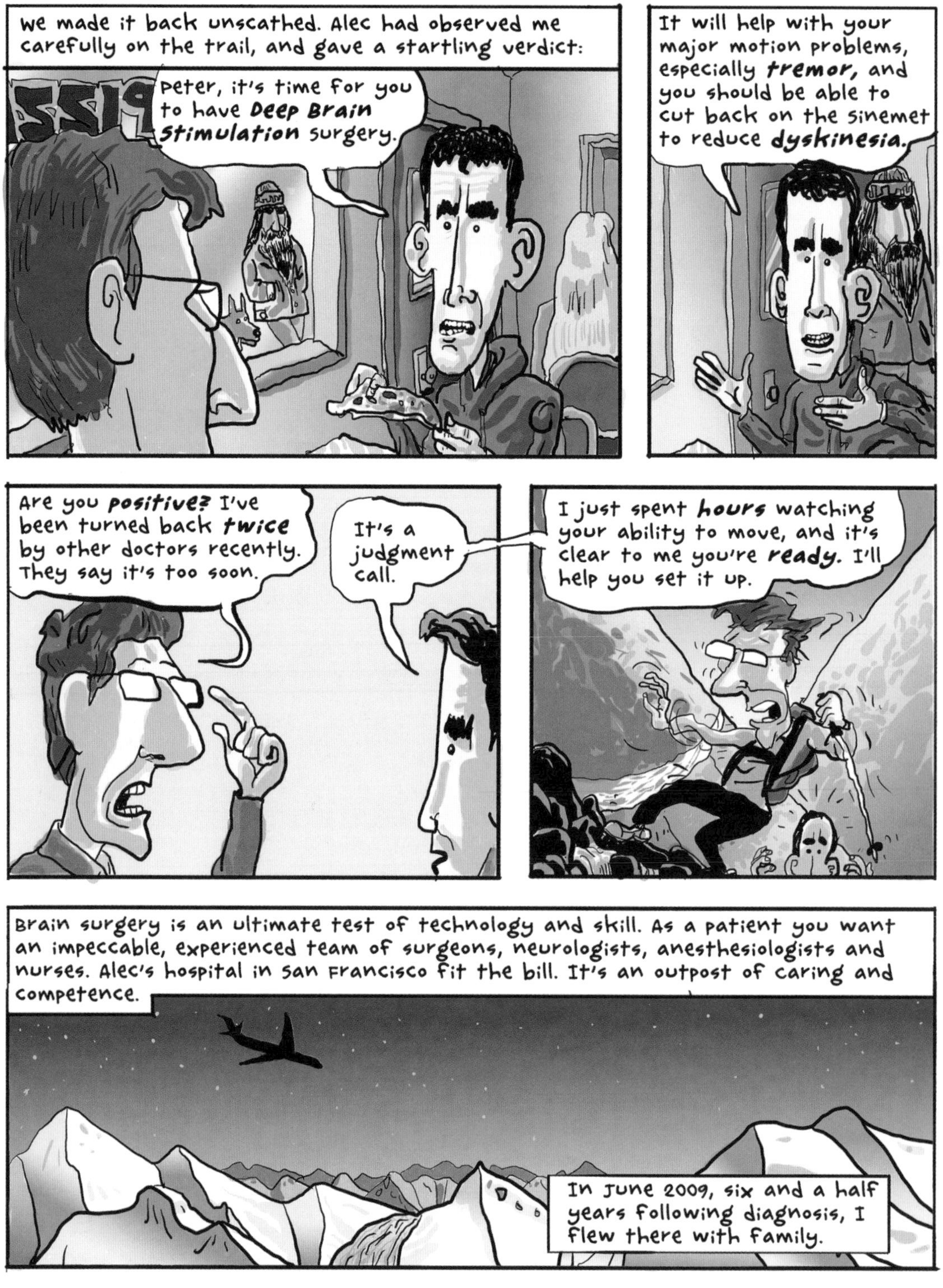
We made it back unscathed. Alec had observed me carefully on the trail, and gave a startling verdict:
Peter, it's time for you to have **Deep Brain Stimulation** surgery.
It will help with your major motion problems, especially **tremor,** and you should be able to cut back on the sinemet to reduce **dyskinesia.**
Are you **positive?** I've been turned back **twice** by other doctors recently. They say it's too soon.
It's a judgment call.
I just spent **hours** watching your ability to move, and it's clear to me you're **ready.** I'll help you set it up.
Brain surgery is an ultimate test of technology and skill. As a patient you want an impeccable, experienced team of surgeons, neurologists, anesthesiologists and nurses. Alec's hospital in San Francisco fit the bill. It's an outpost of caring and competence.
In June 2009, six and a half years following diagnosis, I flew there with family.

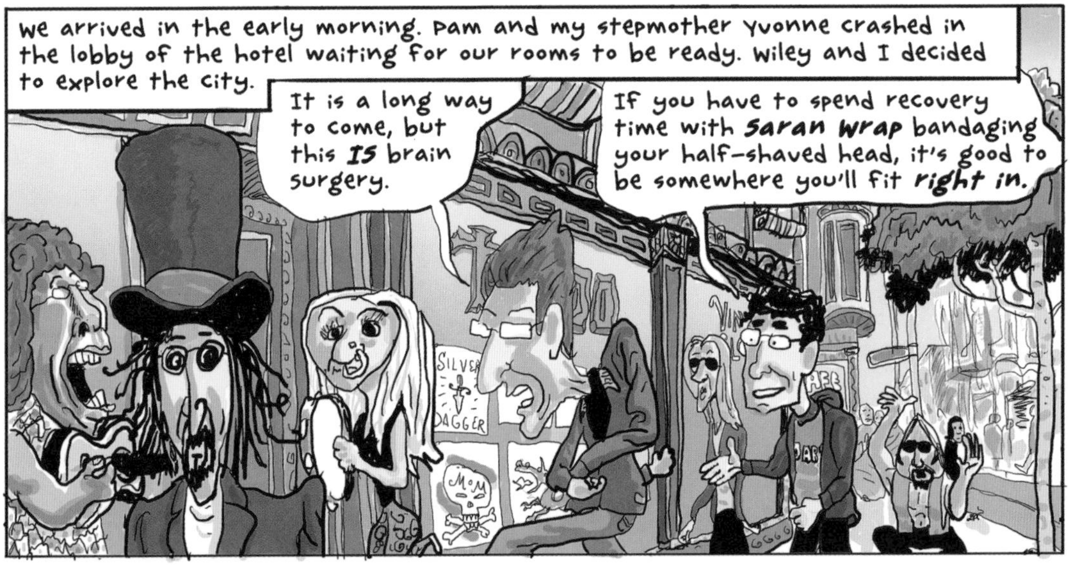
We arrived in the early morning. Pam and my stepmother Yvonne crashed in the lobby of the hotel waiting for our rooms to be ready. Wiley and I decided to explore the city.
It is a long way to come, but this IS brain surgery.
If you have to spend recovery time with Saran Wrap bandaging your half-shaved head, it's good to be somewhere you'll fit right in.
SILVER DAGGER

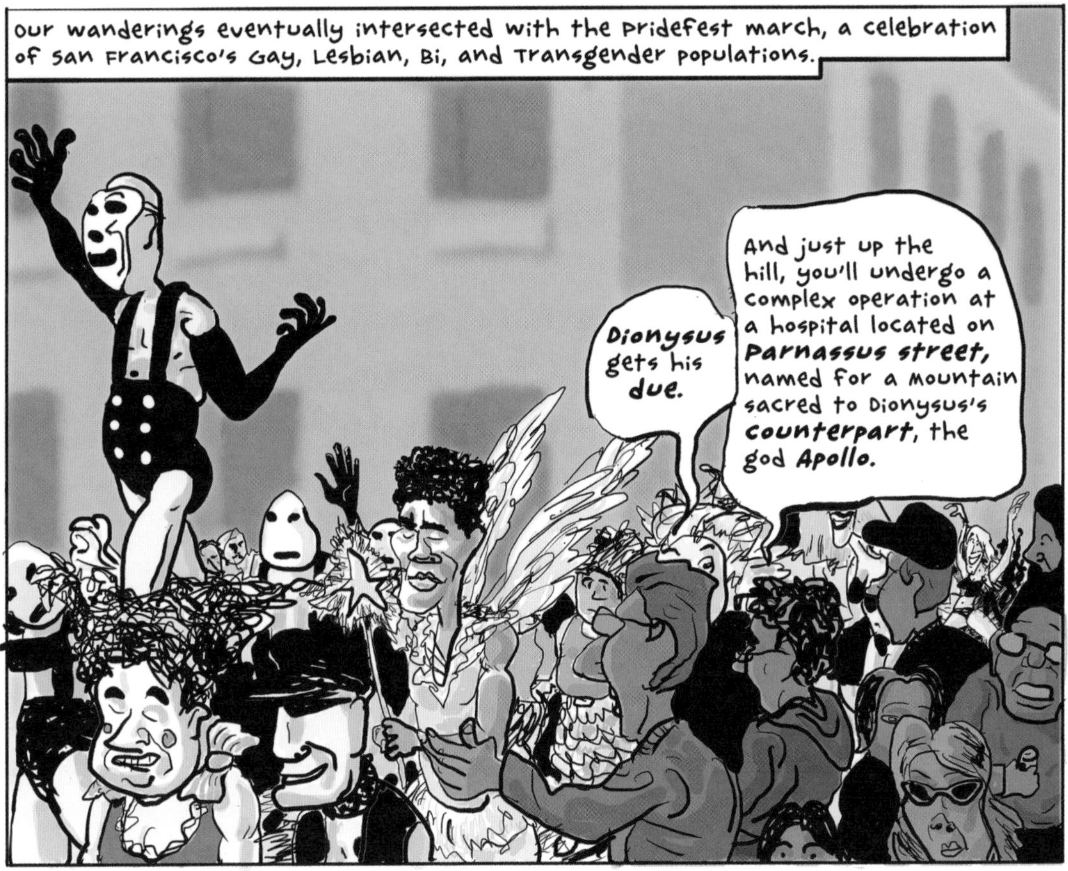
Our wanderings eventually intersected with the Pridefest march, a celebration of San Francisco's Gay, Lesbian, Bi, and Transgender populations.
Dionysus gets his due.
And just up the hill, you'll undergo a complex operation at a hospital located on Parnassus Street, named for a mountain sacred to Dionysus's counterpart, the god Apollo.

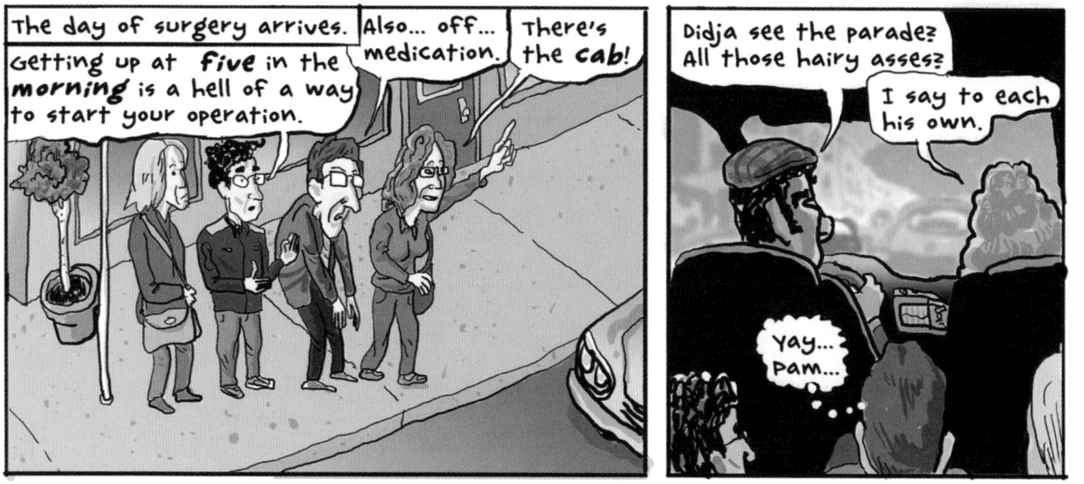
The day of surgery arrives.
Getting up at *five* in the *morning* is a hell of a way to start your operation.
Also... off... medication.
There's the *cab*!
Didja see the parade? All those hairy asses?
I say to each his own.
Yay... Pam...

DEEP BRAIN STIMULATION: the "pacemaker for the brain"

1.) "Deep Brain" means the inner area near the base of the brain. This region of the brain holds a small structure that becomes overactive in PD patients and inhibits motion. The DBS team bores a hole in the patient's skull and passes the lead, an insulated wire with four contact points along its length, to the target structure. This can be done on either or both sides of a brain, depending on symptoms.

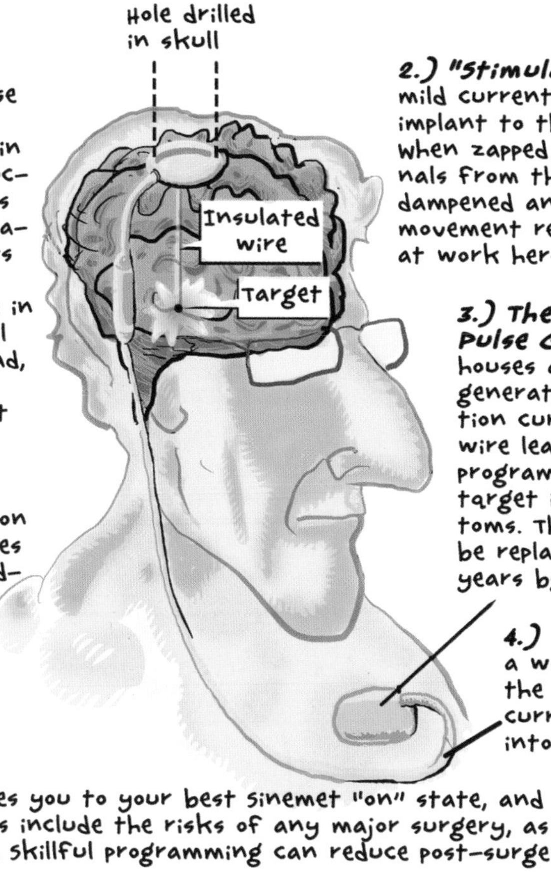
Hole drilled in skull
Insulated wire
Target

2.) "Stimulation" refers to a mild current carried on the wire implant to the target structure. When zapped with the charge, signals from the structure are dampened and significantly freer movement results. The mechanism at work here is poorly understood.

3.) The Implanted Pulse Generator (IPG) houses a battery that generates the stimulation current for the wire lead. The IPG can be programmed to custom-target individual symptoms. The battery must be replaced every few years by a surgeon.

4.) The extension is a wire tunneled under the skin to carry current from the IPG into the brain.

DBS ideally restores you to your best Sinemet "on" state, and makes it last longer. Possible downsides include the risks of any major surgery, as well as speech and balance problems. Skillful programming can reduce post-surgery problems.

The surgery begins with a ritual of faith.

What could be more symbolic of vulnerability and hope than taking off everyday clothes...

...and donning the uniform of a patient?

Just before the drilling starts, the surgeon, Dr. Starr, hands me one last bit of paperwork.

This form says that you have no **moral objection** to a blood transfusion should you need it.

That would be my position.

I have a moral objection to **not** having one if I need it.

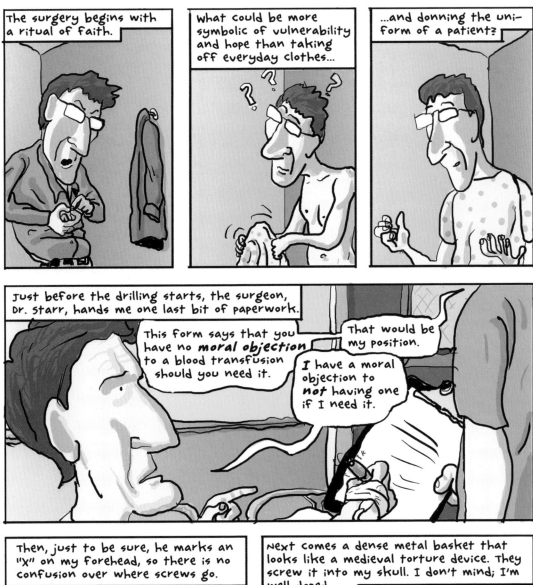

Then, just to be sure, he marks an "X" on my forehead, so there is no confusion over where screws go.

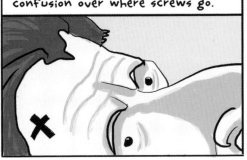

Next comes a dense metal basket that looks like a medieval torture device. They screw it into my skull. I don't mind; I'm well doped.

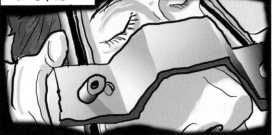

All fades to black. The frame is locked down, immobilizing my head. This assures the precision of the lead placement. The front half of my scalp is shaved. Drilling begins.

The lead is eased in. The team wakes me to gauge my response to the wire's position. They follow a map made from a composite of an MRI and a CAT scan.

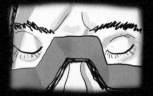 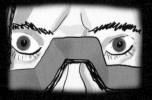

The team is also listening for the telltale sound made by the particular cells they are after. I listen, too, and am disappointed to find that my brain sounds like static on the radio. But maybe that static is more than we know...

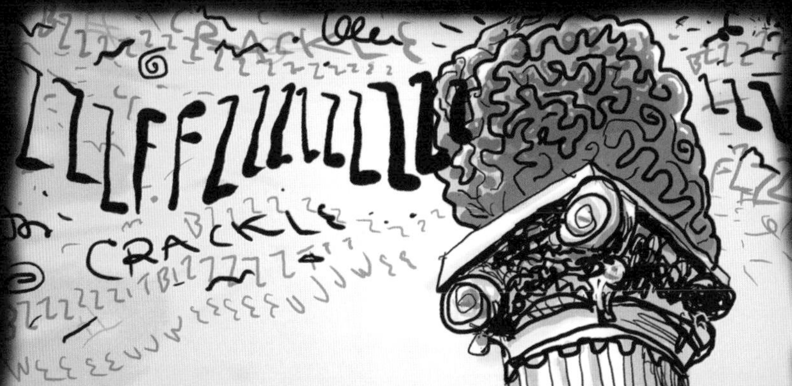

...maybe your radio is bringing you the sounds of the neurons of the deep brain of God... **WHOA.** I **am** well medicated!

I have no pain from the wire. The brain does not feel injury to itself. Normally if there is a foreign object in your brain, you are beyond help, so there is no purpose to processing it as pain.

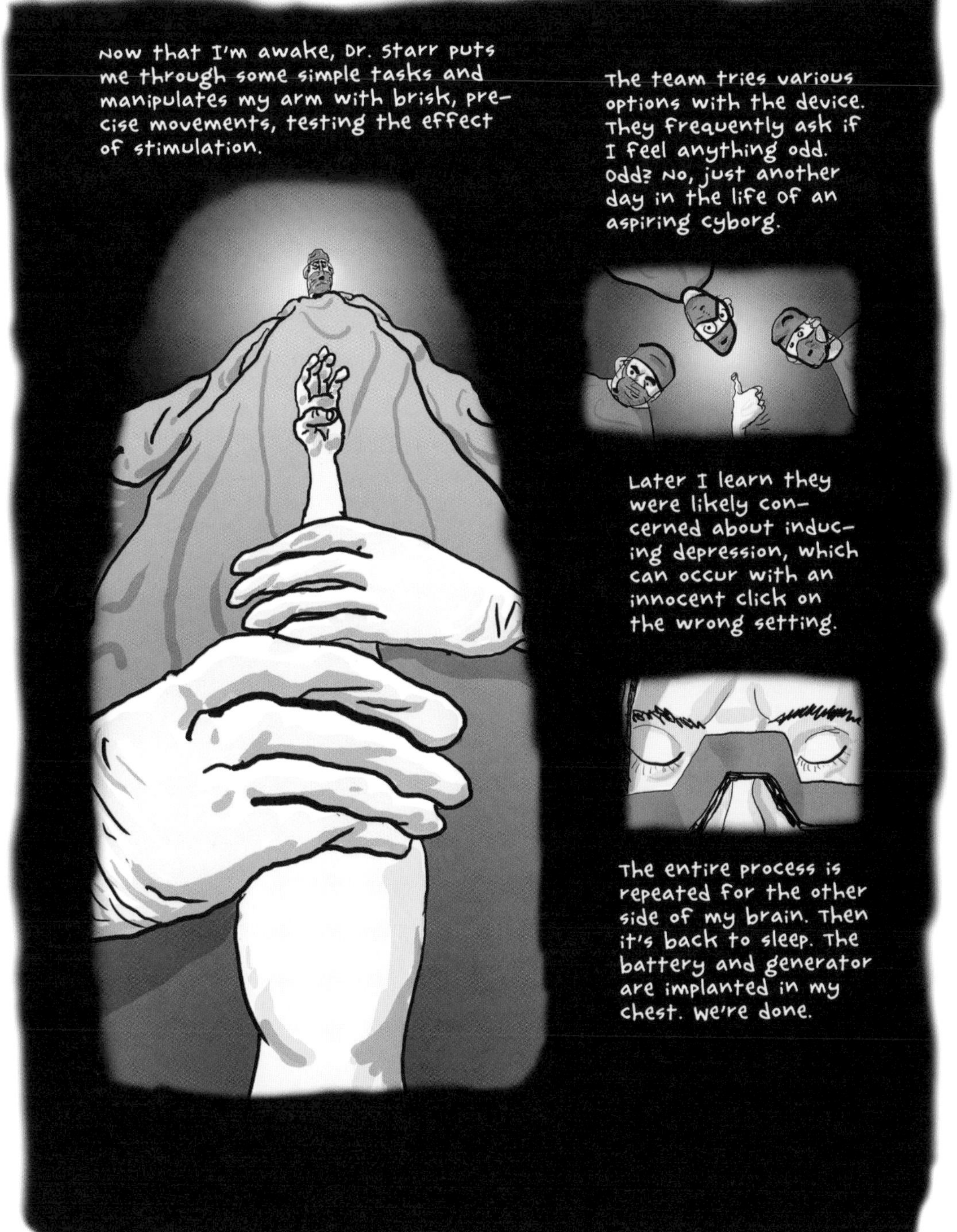
Now that I'm awake, Dr. Starr puts me through some simple tasks and manipulates my arm with brisk, precise movements, testing the effect of stimulation.
The team tries various options with the device. They frequently ask if I feel anything odd. Odd? No, just another day in the life of an aspiring cyborg.
Later I learn they were likely concerned about inducing depression, which can occur with an innocent click on the wrong setting.
The entire process is repeated for the other side of my brain. Then it's back to sleep. The battery and generator are implanted in my chest. We're done.

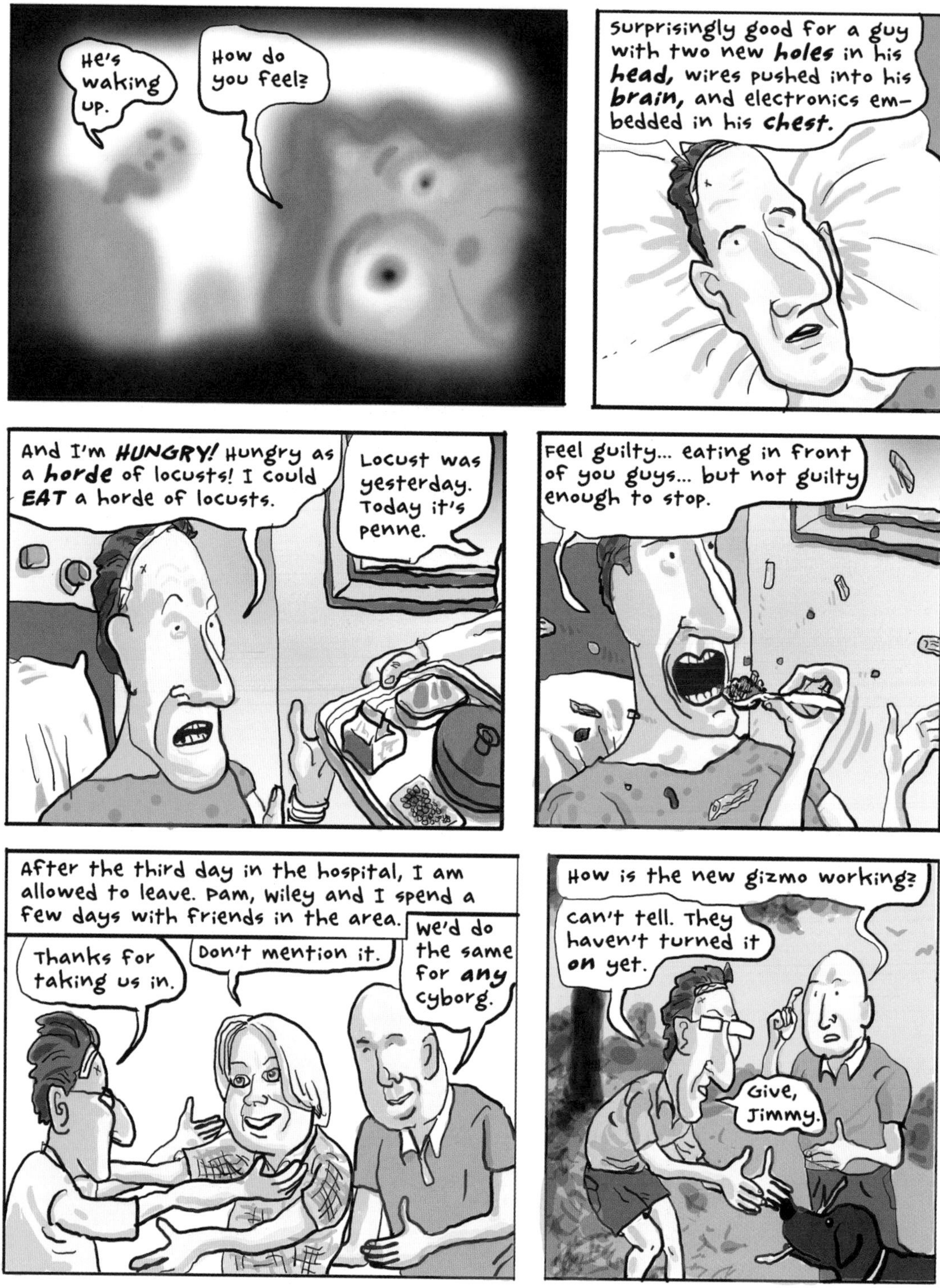
He's waking up.
How do you feel?
Surprisingly good for a guy with two new holes in his head, wires pushed into his brain, and electronics embedded in his chest.
And I'm HUNGRY! Hungry as a horde of locusts! I could EAT a horde of locusts.
Locust was yesterday. Today it's penne.
Feel guilty... eating in front of you guys... but not guilty enough to stop.
After the third day in the hospital, I am allowed to leave. Pam, Wiley and I spend a few days with friends in the area.
Thanks for taking us in.
Don't mention it.
We'd do the same for any cyborg.
How is the new gizmo working?
Can't tell. They haven't turned it on yet.
Give, Jimmy.

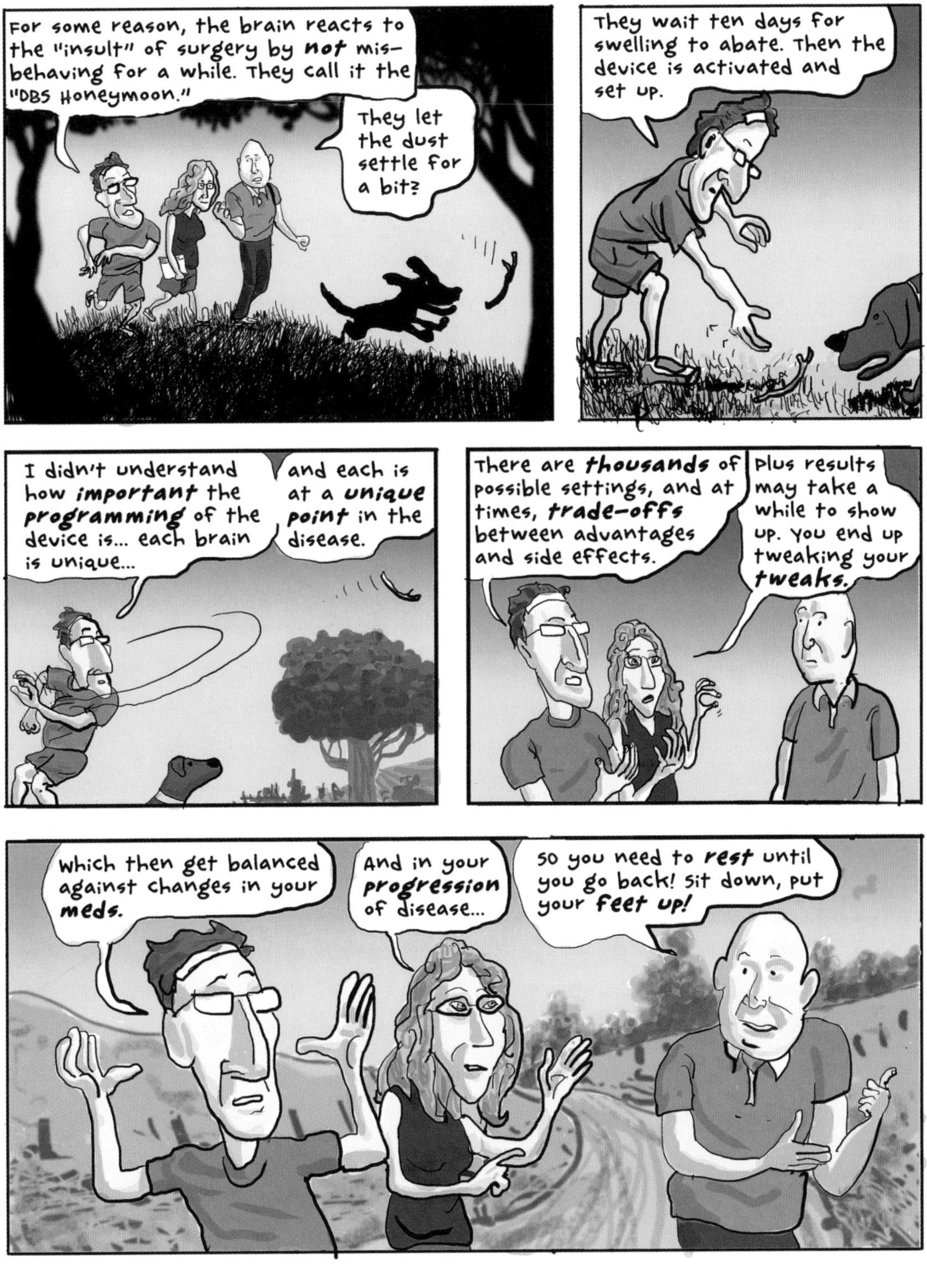

For some reason, the brain reacts to the "insult" of surgery by **not** misbehaving for a while. They call it the "DBS Honeymoon."
They let the dust settle for a bit?
They wait ten days for swelling to abate. Then the device is activated and set up.
I didn't understand how **important** the **programming** of the device is... each brain is unique...
and each is at a **unique point** in the disease.
There are **thousands** of possible settings, and at times, **trade-offs** between advantages and side effects.
Plus results may take a while to show up. You end up tweaking your **tweaks.**
Which then get balanced against changes in your **meds.**
And in your **progression** of disease...
So you need to **rest** until you go back! Sit down, put your **feet up!**

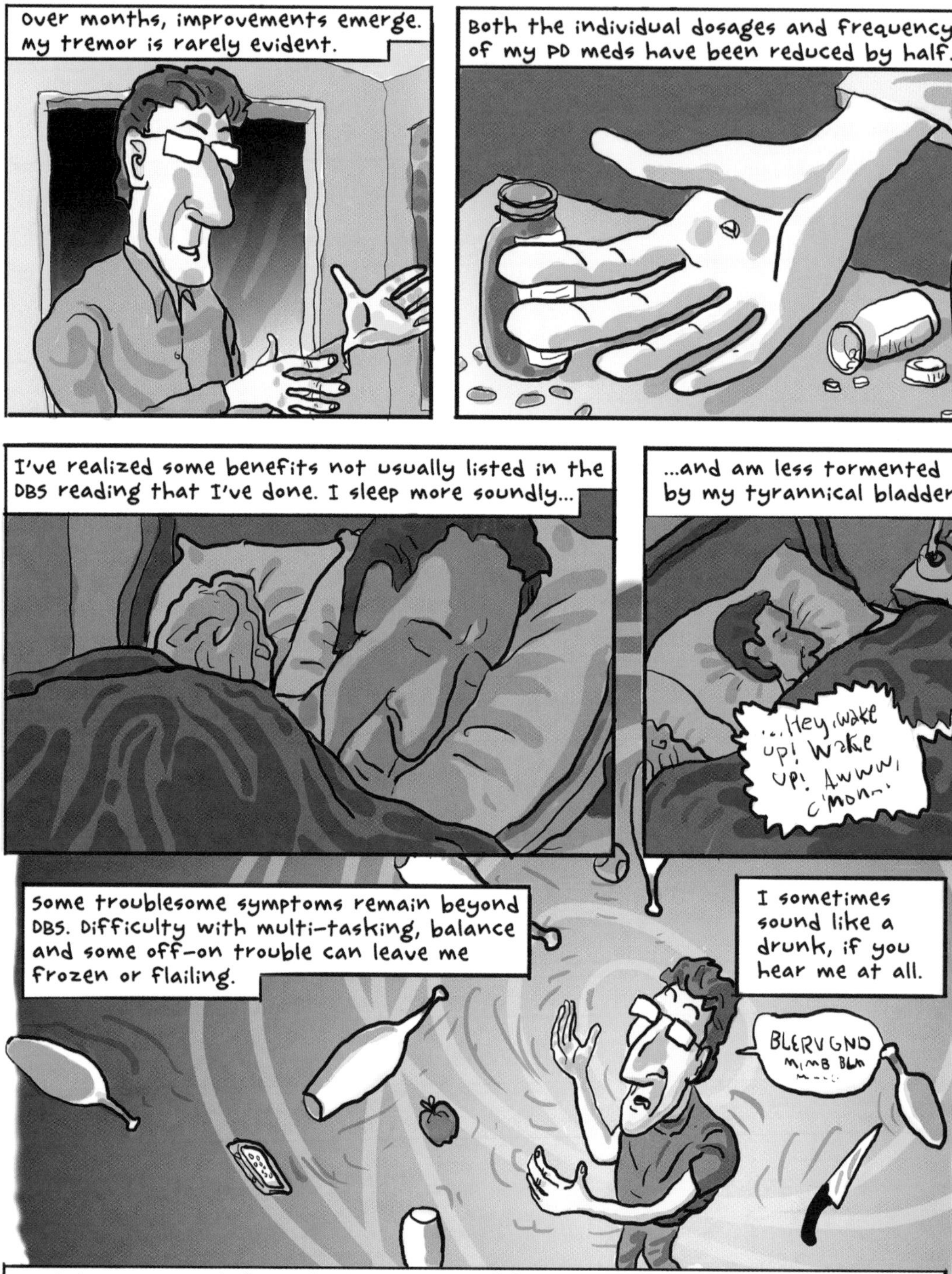
Over months, improvements emerge. My tremor is rarely evident.
Both the individual dosages and frequency of my PD meds have been reduced by half.
I've realized some benefits not usually listed in the DBS reading that I've done. I sleep more soundly...
...and am less tormented by my tyrannical bladder.
...Hey, wake up! Wake up! Awww, c'mon...
Some troublesome symptoms remain beyond DBS. Difficulty with multi-tasking, balance and some off-on trouble can leave me frozen or flailing.
I sometimes sound like a drunk, if you hear me at all.
BLERVGND MIMB BLA
...But ten years out from diagnosis I'm still buttoning my own shirt, cutting my own food, riding my bike, and exploring the Island of the caring and competent.

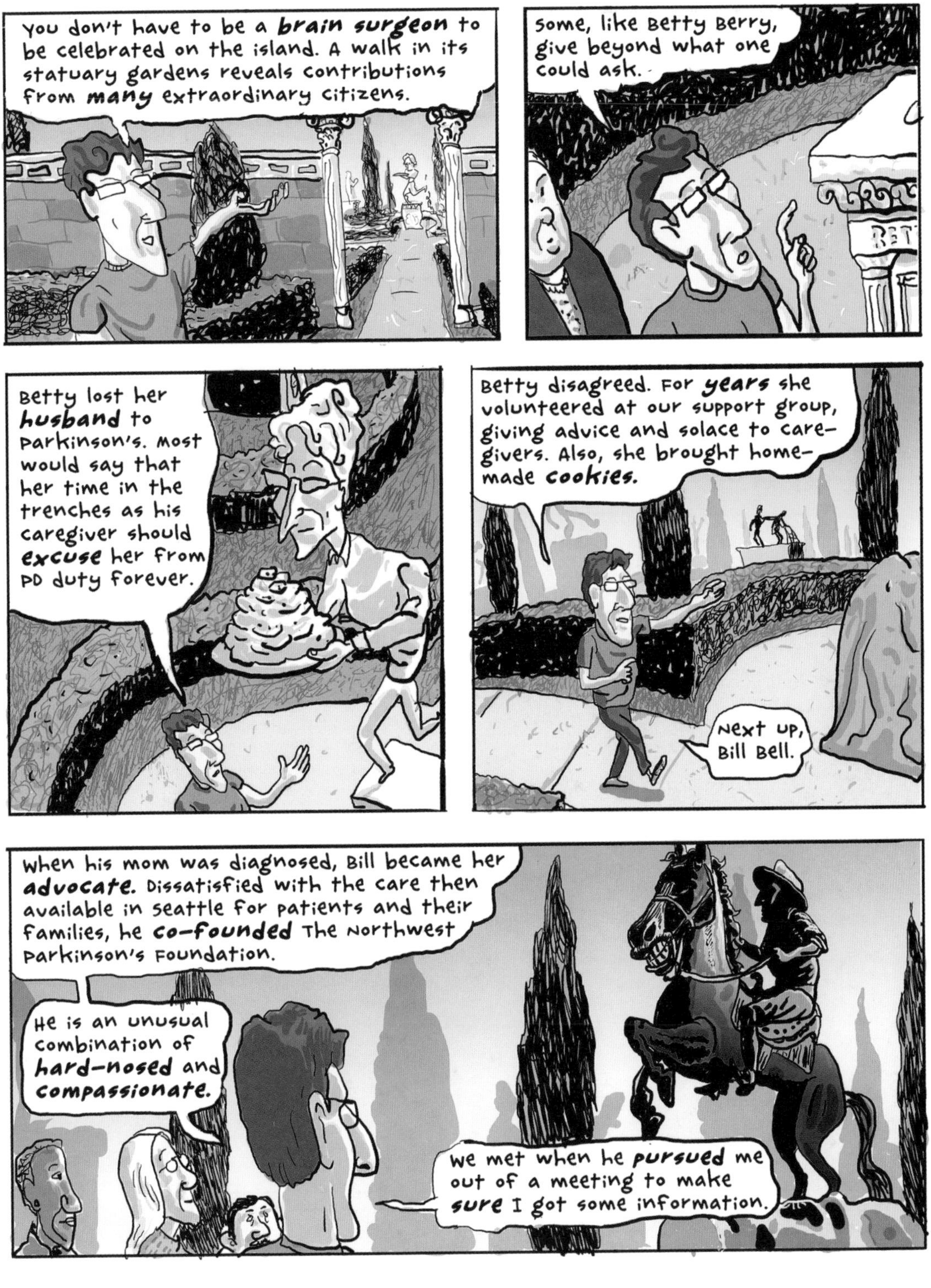
You don't have to be a brain surgeon to be celebrated on the island. A walk in its statuary gardens reveals contributions from many extraordinary citizens.
Some, like Betty Berry, give beyond what one could ask.
Betty lost her husband to Parkinson's. Most would say that her time in the trenches as his caregiver should excuse her from PD duty forever.
Betty disagreed. For years she volunteered at our support group, giving advice and solace to caregivers. Also, she brought homemade cookies.
Next up, Bill Bell.
When his mom was diagnosed, Bill became her advocate. Dissatisfied with the care then available in Seattle for patients and their families, he co-founded The Northwest Parkinson's Foundation.
He is an unusual combination of hard-nosed and compassionate.
We met when he pursued me out of a meeting to make sure I got some information.

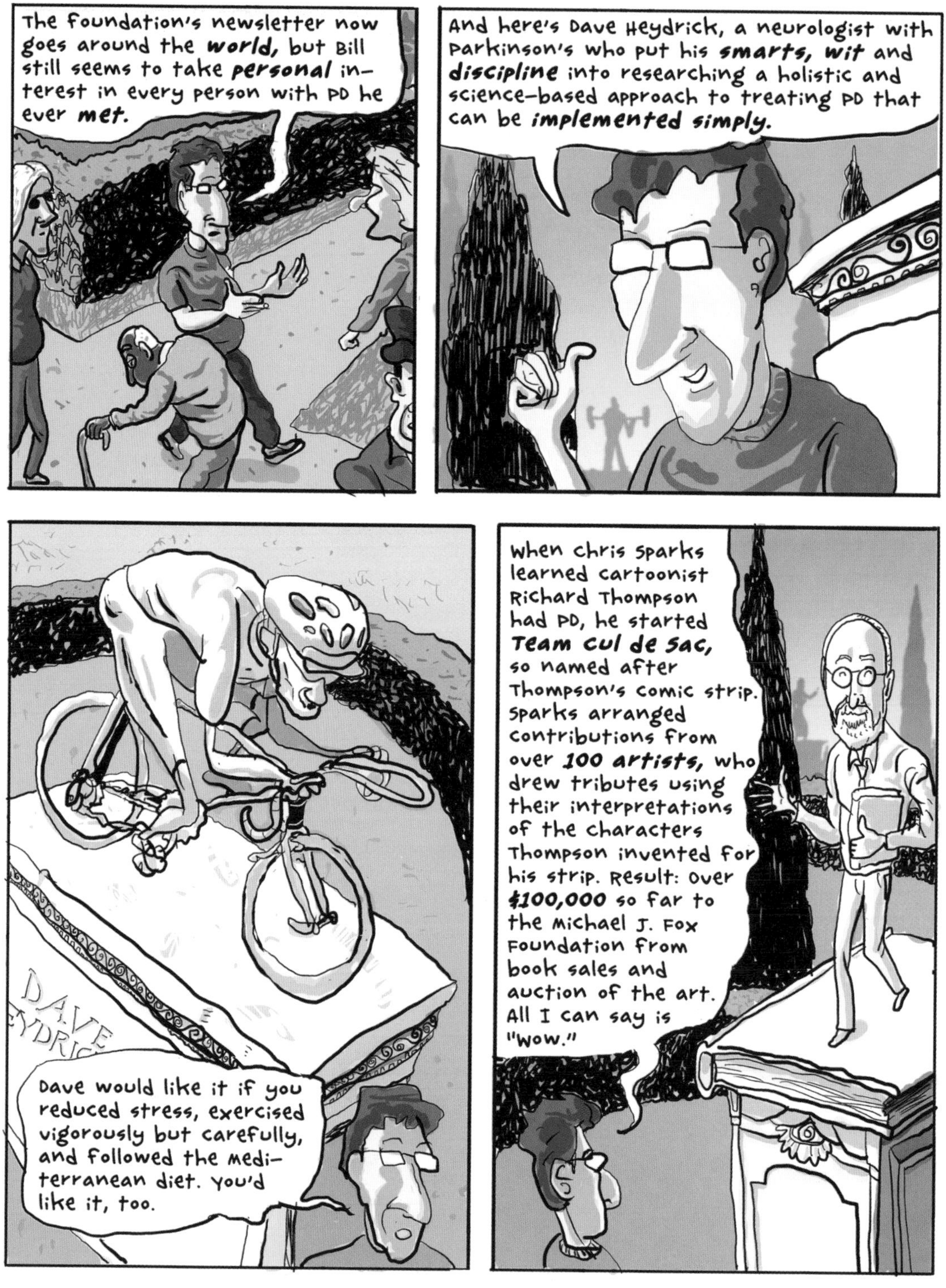
The foundation's newsletter now goes around the **world,** but Bill still seems to take **personal** interest in every person with PD he ever **met.**
And here's Dave Heydrick, a neurologist with Parkinson's who put his **smarts, wit** and **discipline** into researching a holistic and science-based approach to treating PD that can be **implemented simply.**
DAVE HEYDRIC
Dave would like it if you reduced stress, exercised vigorously but carefully, and followed the mediterranean diet. You'd like it, too.
When Chris Sparks learned cartoonist Richard Thompson had PD, he started **Team Cul de Sac,** so named after Thompson's comic strip. Sparks arranged contributions from over **100 artists,** who drew tributes using their interpretations of the characters Thompson invented for his strip. Result: Over **$100,000** so far to the Michael J. Fox Foundation from book sales and auction of the art. All I can say is "Wow."

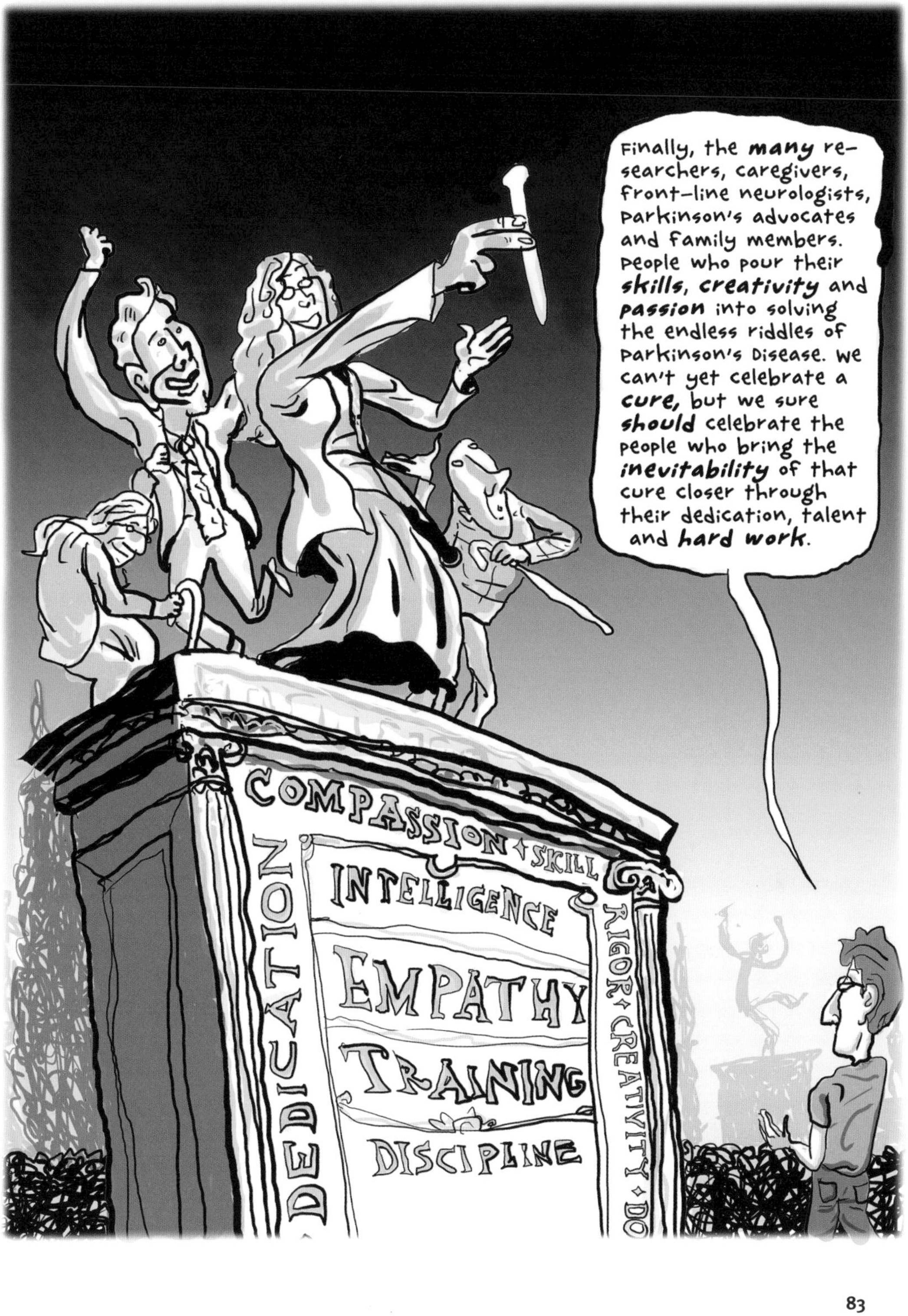
Finally, the **many** researchers, caregivers, front-line neurologists, Parkinson's advocates and family members. People who pour their ***skills, creativity*** and ***passion*** into solving the endless riddles of Parkinson's Disease. We can't yet celebrate a ***cure,*** but we sure ***should*** celebrate the people who bring the ***inevitability*** of that cure closer through their dedication, talent and ***hard work***.
COMPASSION ✦ SKILL
INTELLIGENCE
EMPATHY
TRAINING
DISCIPLINE
DEDICATION
RIGOR ✦ CREATIVITY ✦ DO

7. A Different Path

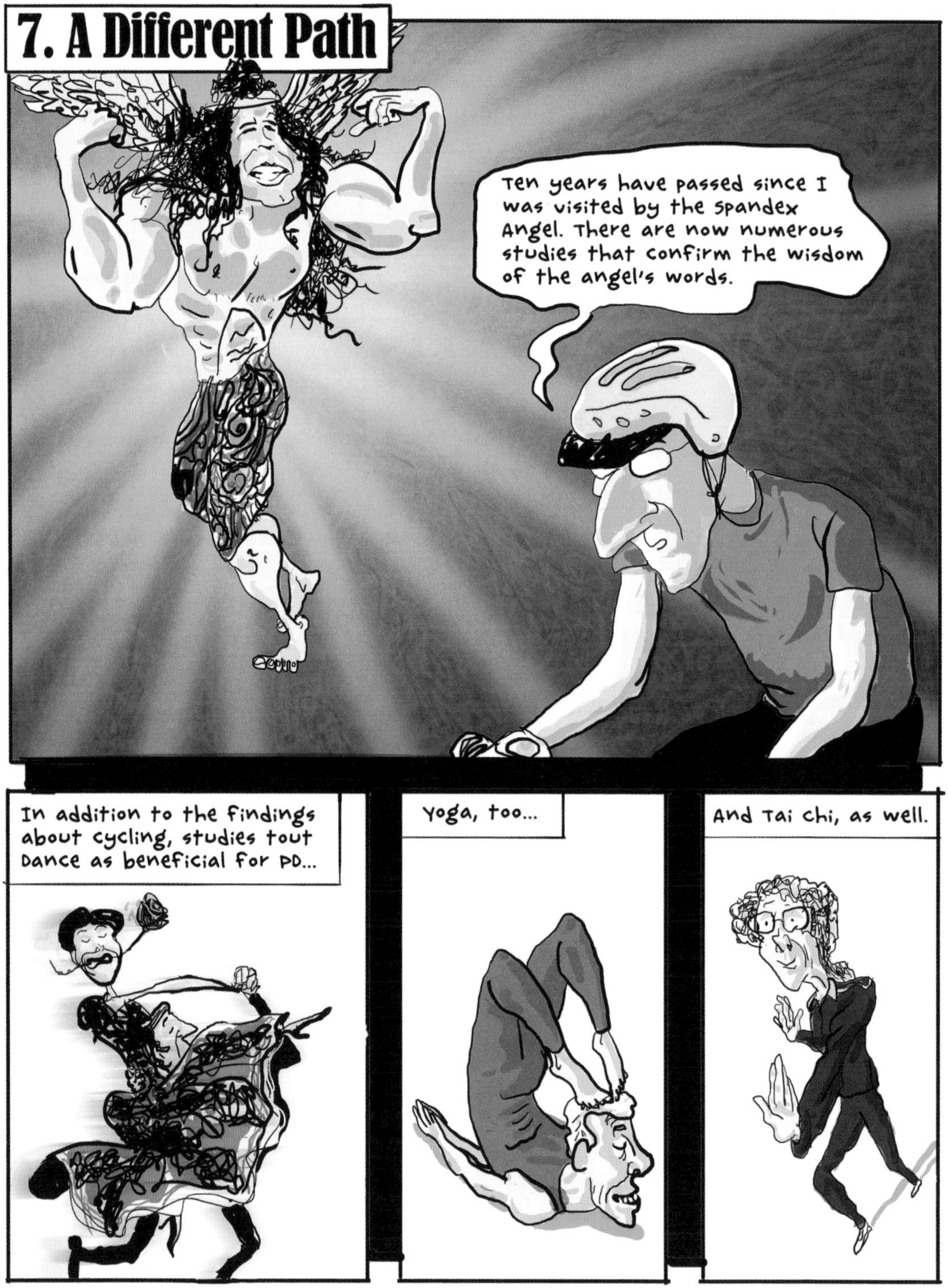
Ten years have passed since I was visited by the spandex Angel. There are now numerous studies that confirm the wisdom of the angel's words.
In addition to the findings about cycling, studies tout Dance as beneficial for PD...
Yoga, too...
And Tai Chi, as well.

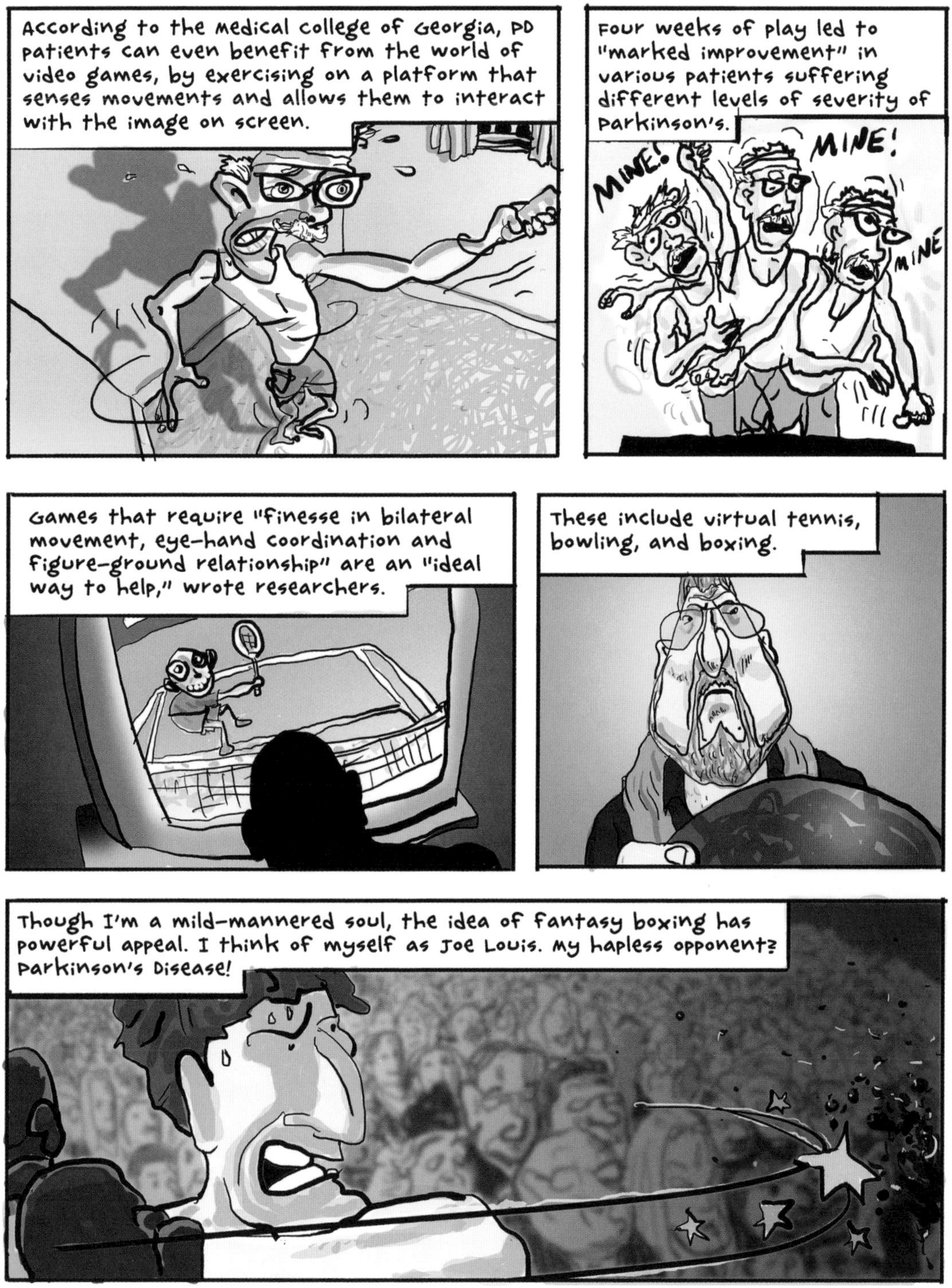
According to the medical college of Georgia, PD patients can even benefit from the world of video games, by exercising on a platform that senses movements and allows them to interact with the image on screen.
Four weeks of play led to "marked improvement" in various patients suffering different levels of severity of Parkinson's.
MINE!
MINE!
MINE
Games that require "finesse in bilateral movement, eye-hand coordination and figure-ground relationship" are an "ideal way to help," wrote researchers.
These include virtual tennis, bowling, and boxing.
Though I'm a mild-mannered soul, the idea of fantasy boxing has powerful appeal. I think of myself as Joe Louis. My hapless opponent? Parkinson's Disease!

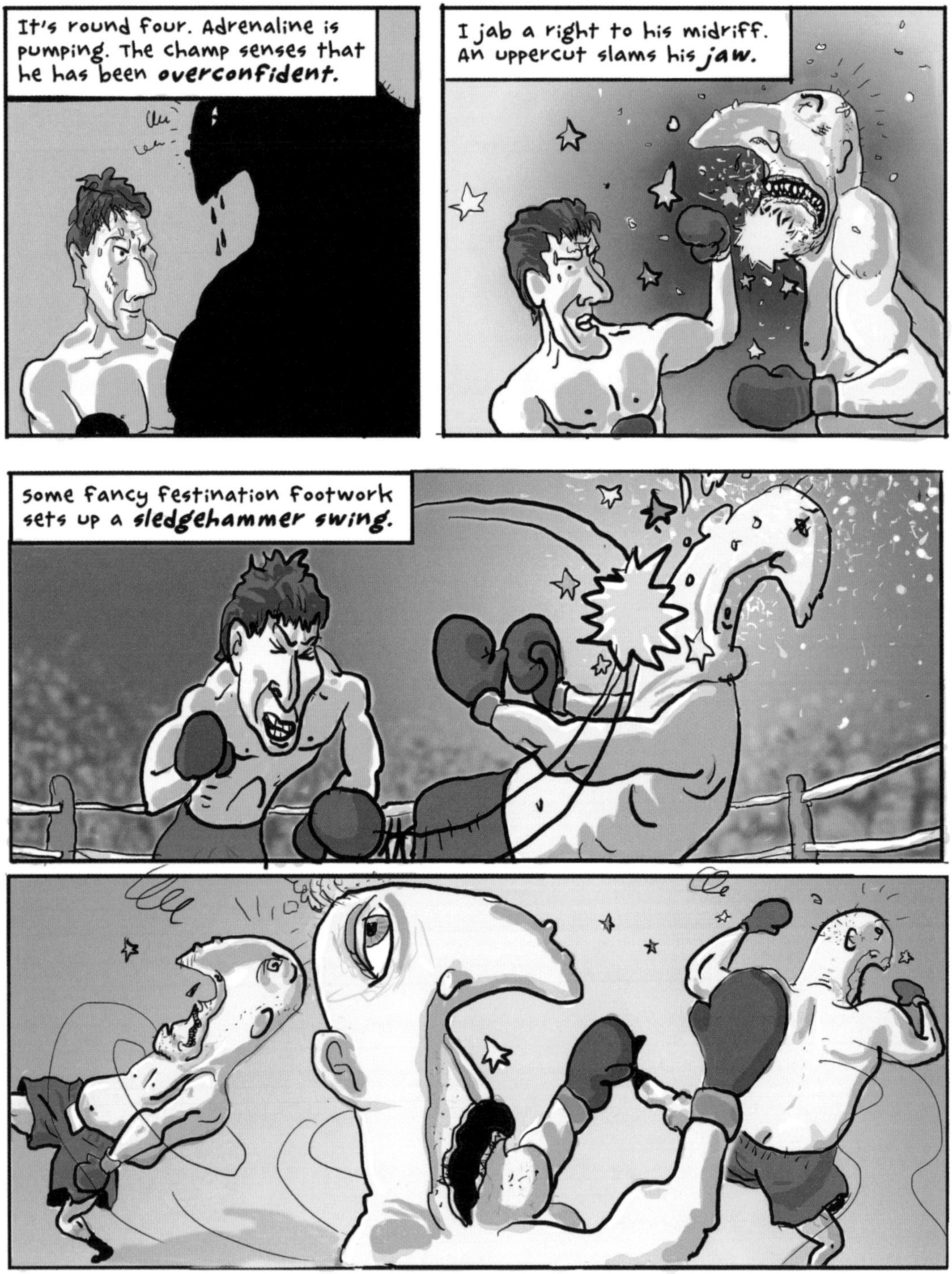
It's round four. Adrenaline is pumping. The champ senses that he has been overconfident.
I jab a right to his midriff. An uppercut slams his jaw.
Some fancy festination footwork sets up a sledgehammer swing.

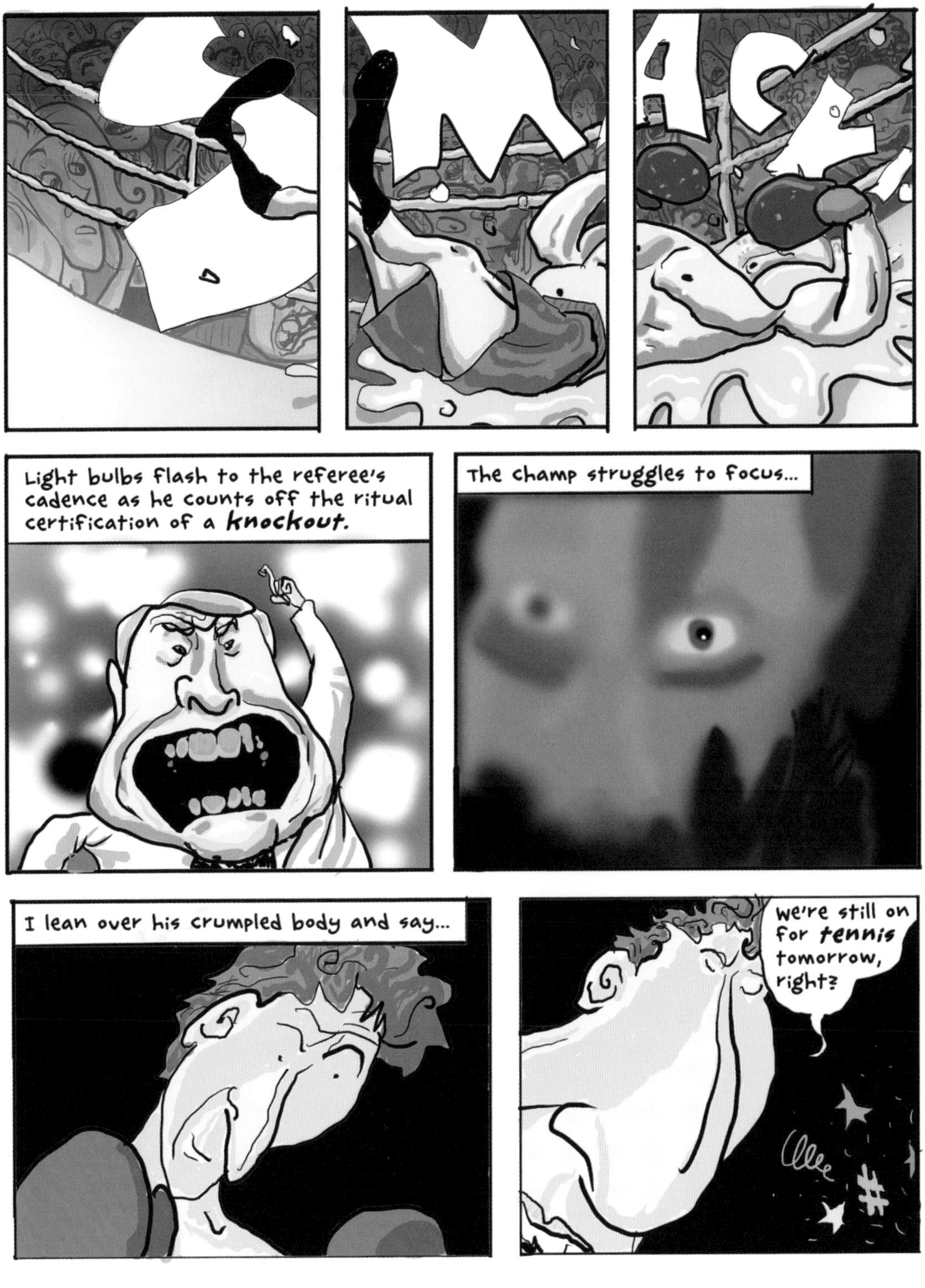
Light bulbs flash to the referee's cadence as he counts off the ritual certification of a knockout.
The champ struggles to focus...
I lean over his crumpled body and say...
We're still on for tennis tomorrow, right?

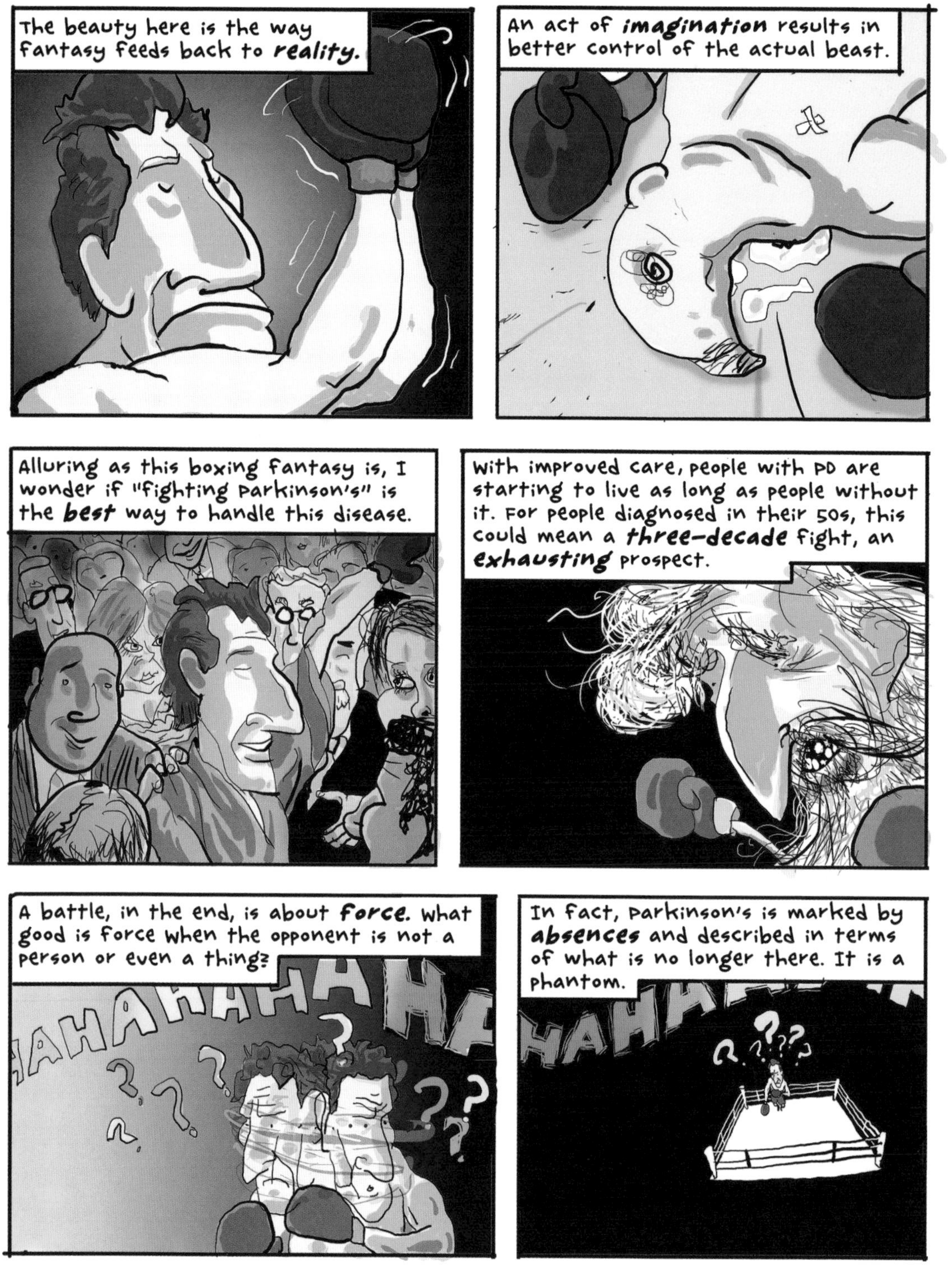

The beauty here is the way fantasy feeds back to *reality.*
An act of *imagination* results in better control of the actual beast.
Alluring as this boxing fantasy is, I wonder if "fighting Parkinson's" is the *best* way to handle this disease.
With improved care, people with PD are starting to live as long as people without it. For people diagnosed in their 50s, this could mean a *three-decade* fight, an *exhausting* prospect.
A battle, in the end, is about *force.* What good is force when the opponent is not a person or even a thing?
HAHAHAHAHA
In fact, Parkinson's is marked by *absences* and described in terms of what is no longer there. It is a phantom.
HAHAHA

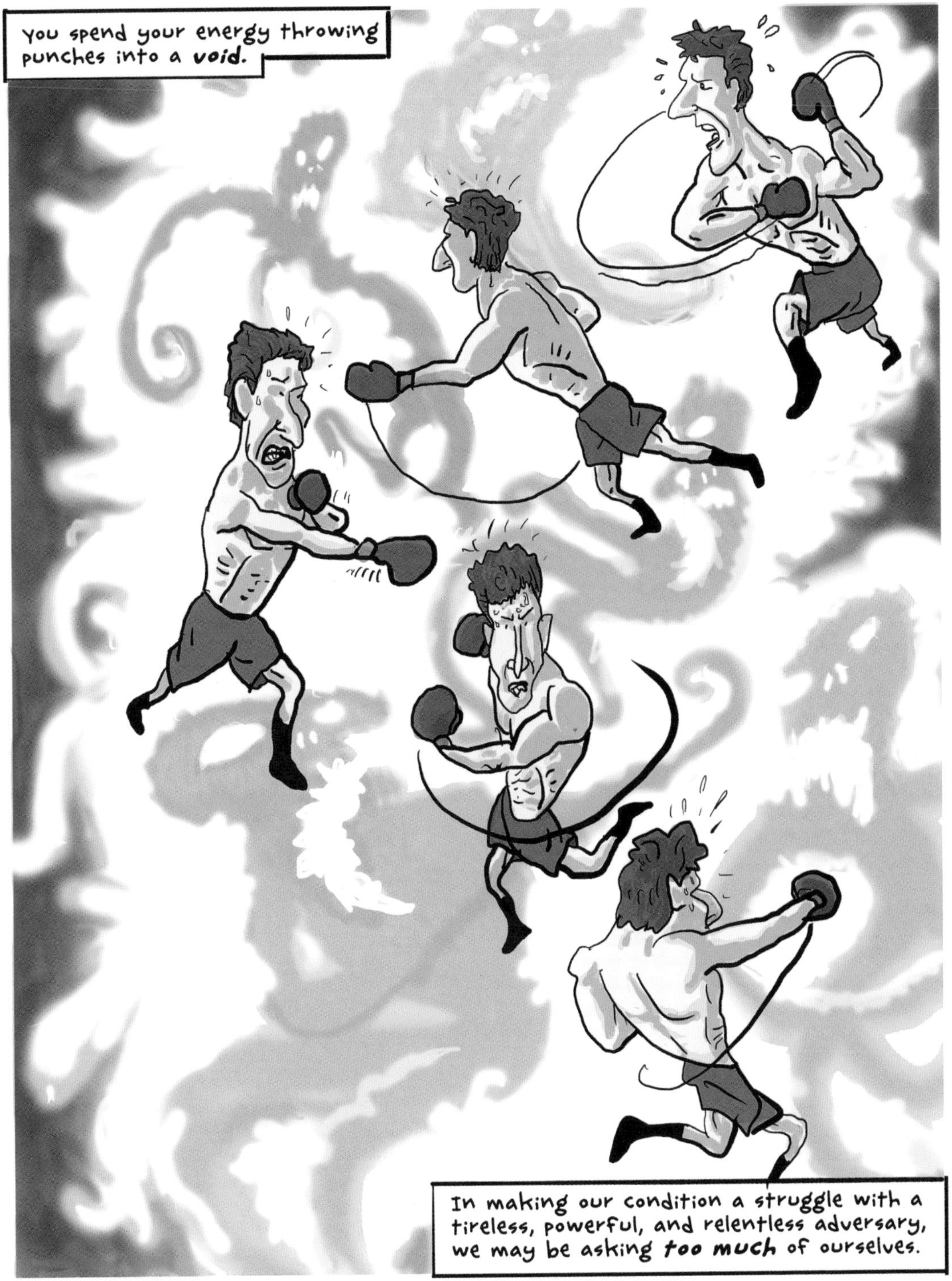
you spend your energy throwing punches into a void.
In making our condition a struggle with a tireless, powerful, and relentless adversary, we may be asking too much of ourselves.

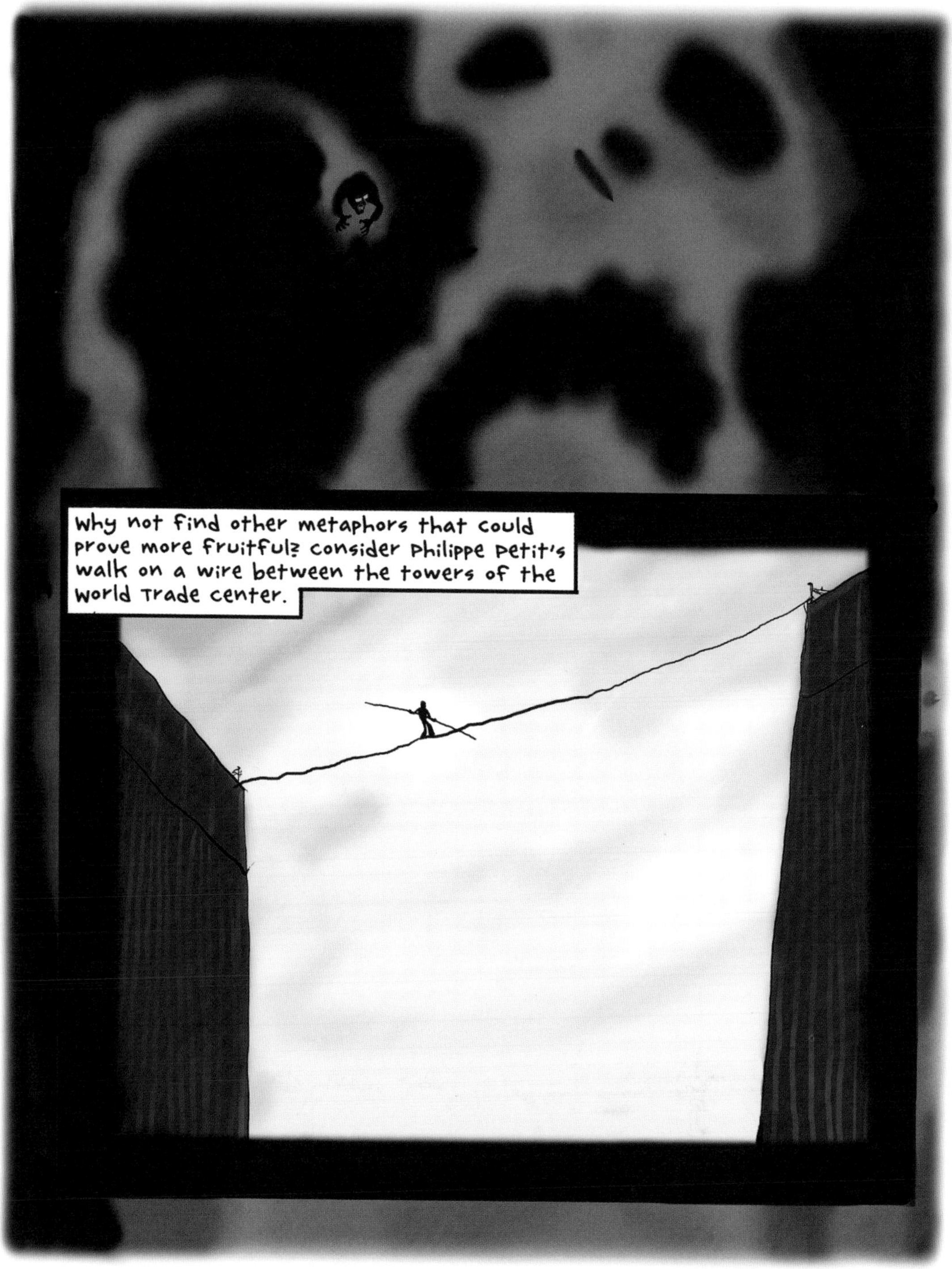
Why not find other metaphors that could prove more fruitful? Consider Philippe Petit's walk on a wire between the towers of the World Trade Center.

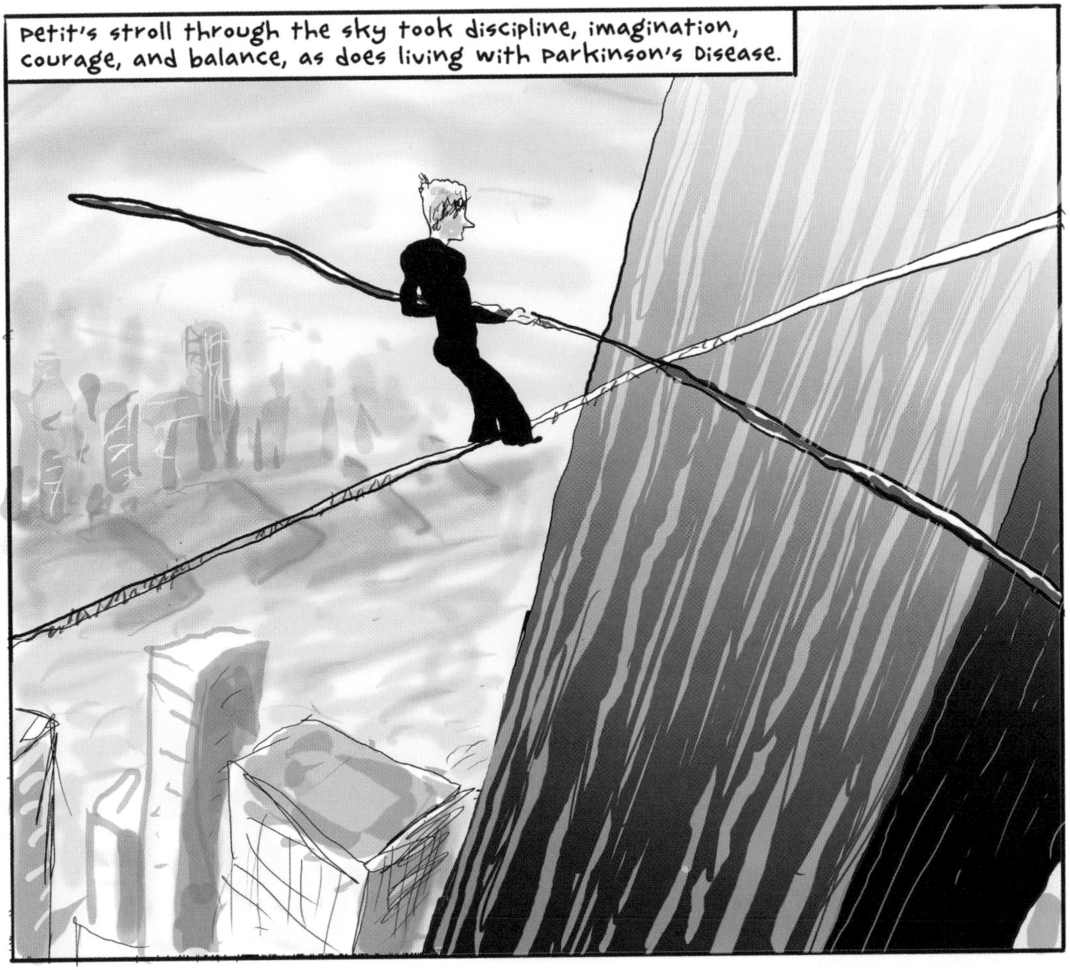
Petit's stroll through the sky took discipline, imagination, courage, and balance, as does living with Parkinson's Disease.

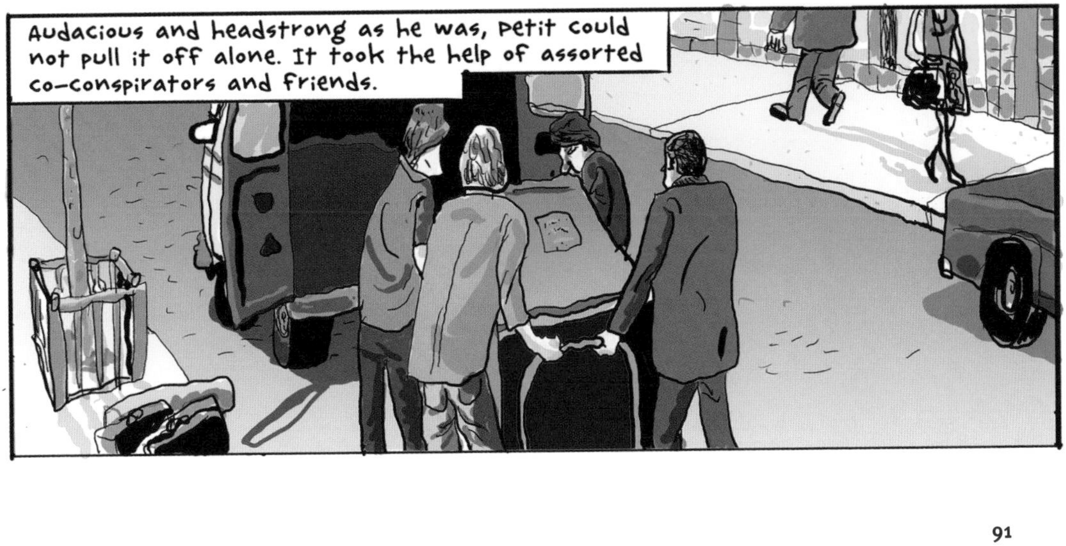
Audacious and headstrong as he was, Petit could not pull it off alone. It took the help of assorted co-conspirators and friends.

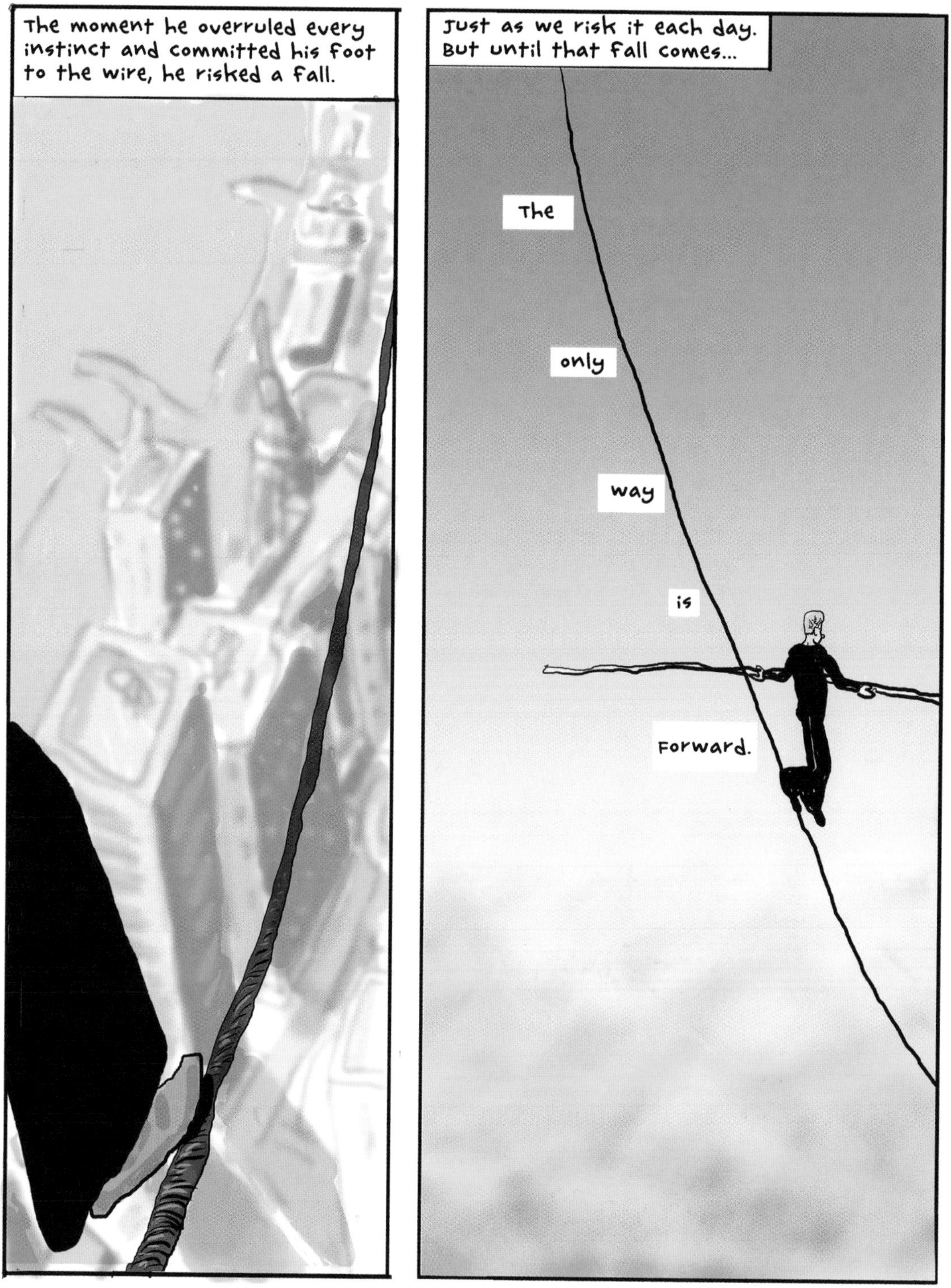
The moment he overruled every instinct and committed his foot to the wire, he risked a fall.
Just as we risk it each day. But until that fall comes...
The
only
way
is
forward.

8. Diagnosis, Reprise

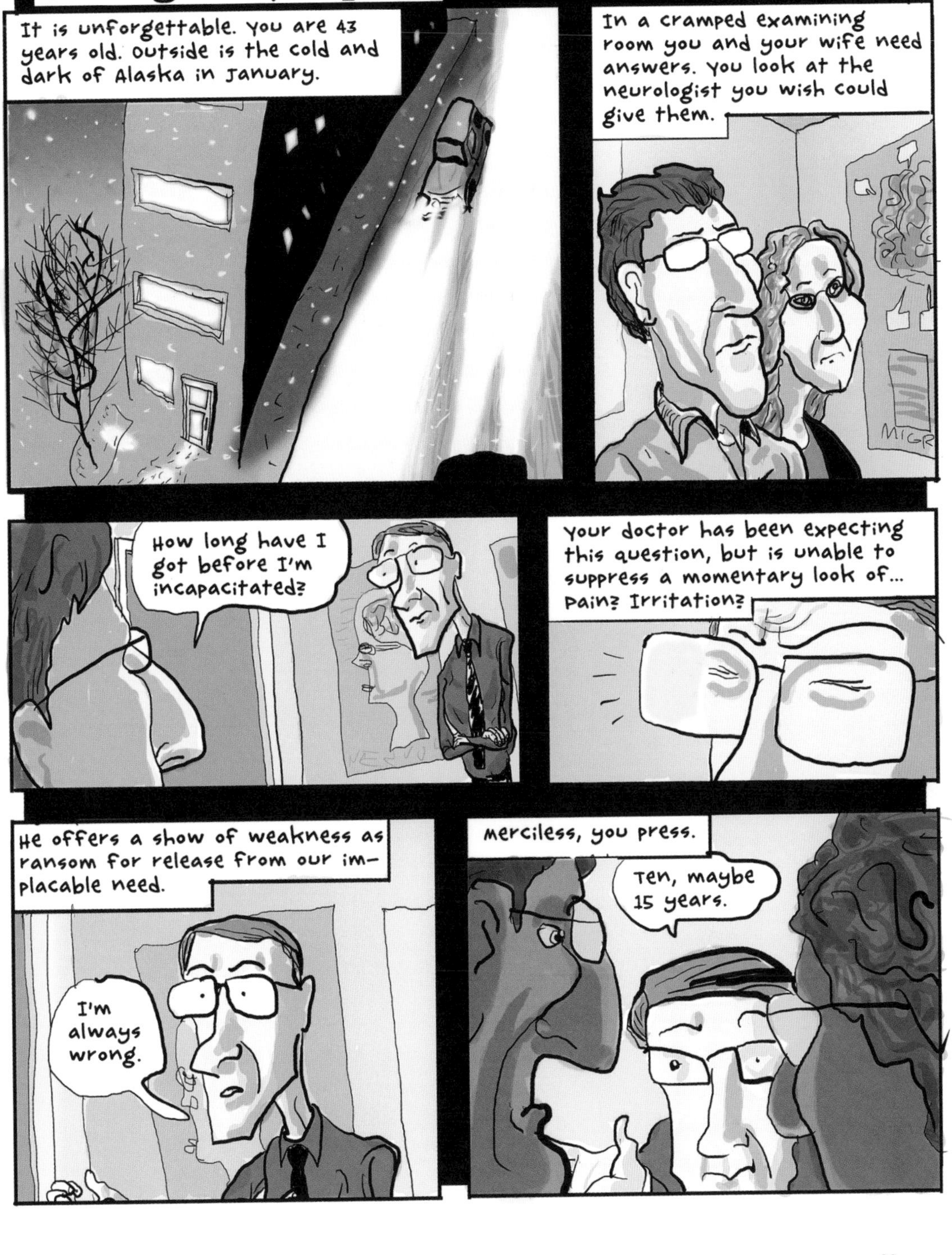
It is unforgettable. You are 43 years old. Outside is the cold and dark of Alaska in January.
In a cramped examining room you and your wife need answers. You look at the neurologist you wish could give them.
MIGR
How long have I got before I'm incapacitated?
Your doctor has been expecting this question, but is unable to suppress a momentary look of... Pain? Irritation?
He offers a show of weakness as ransom for release from our implacable need.
I'm always wrong.
Merciless, you press.
Ten, maybe 15 years.

Ten years? A quick calculation instantly yields a goal. You want to see your son earn his degree from college.

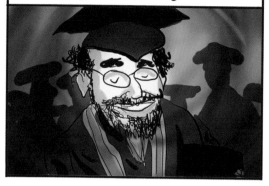

That time seems impossibly distant, the path steep and cut with streams washing it from under your feet.

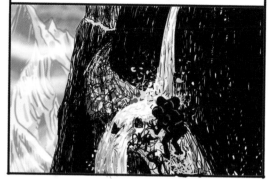

You shoulder your pills, your fears, your responsibilities and your hopes, strike up a dirge, and begin the climb.

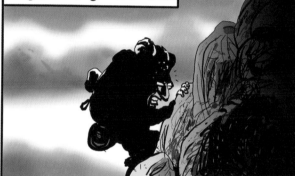

To your great surprise, with the help of many hands, that day arrives in brilliant sunlight. So you will celebrate.

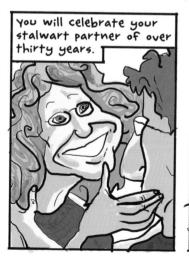

You will celebrate your formidable son, who has graduated with honors in a demanding field.

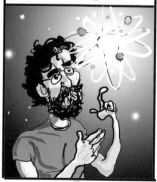

You will celebrate your stalwart partner of over thirty years.

You will celebrate the generosity of family members who come to be with you in this moment of reprieve from the inevitability of loss.

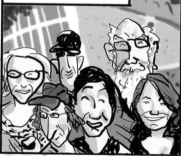

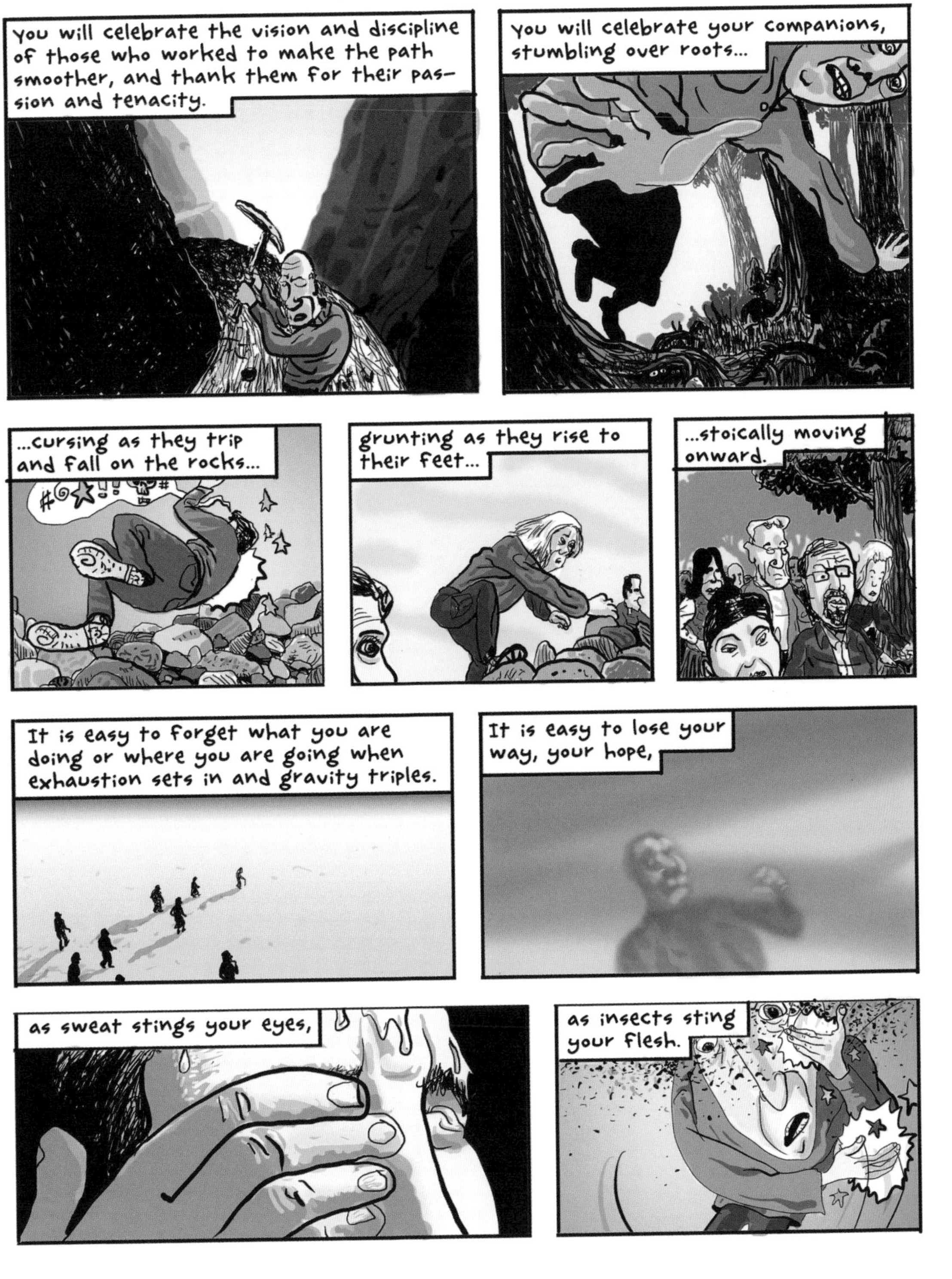
You will celebrate the vision and discipline of those who worked to make the path smoother, and thank them for their passion and tenacity.
You will celebrate your companions, stumbling over roots...
...cursing as they trip and fall on the rocks...
#@☆!!!☠#
grunting as they rise to their feet...
...stoically moving onward.
It is easy to forget what you are doing or where you are going when exhaustion sets in and gravity triples.
It is easy to lose your way, your hope,
as sweat stings your eyes,
as insects sting your flesh.

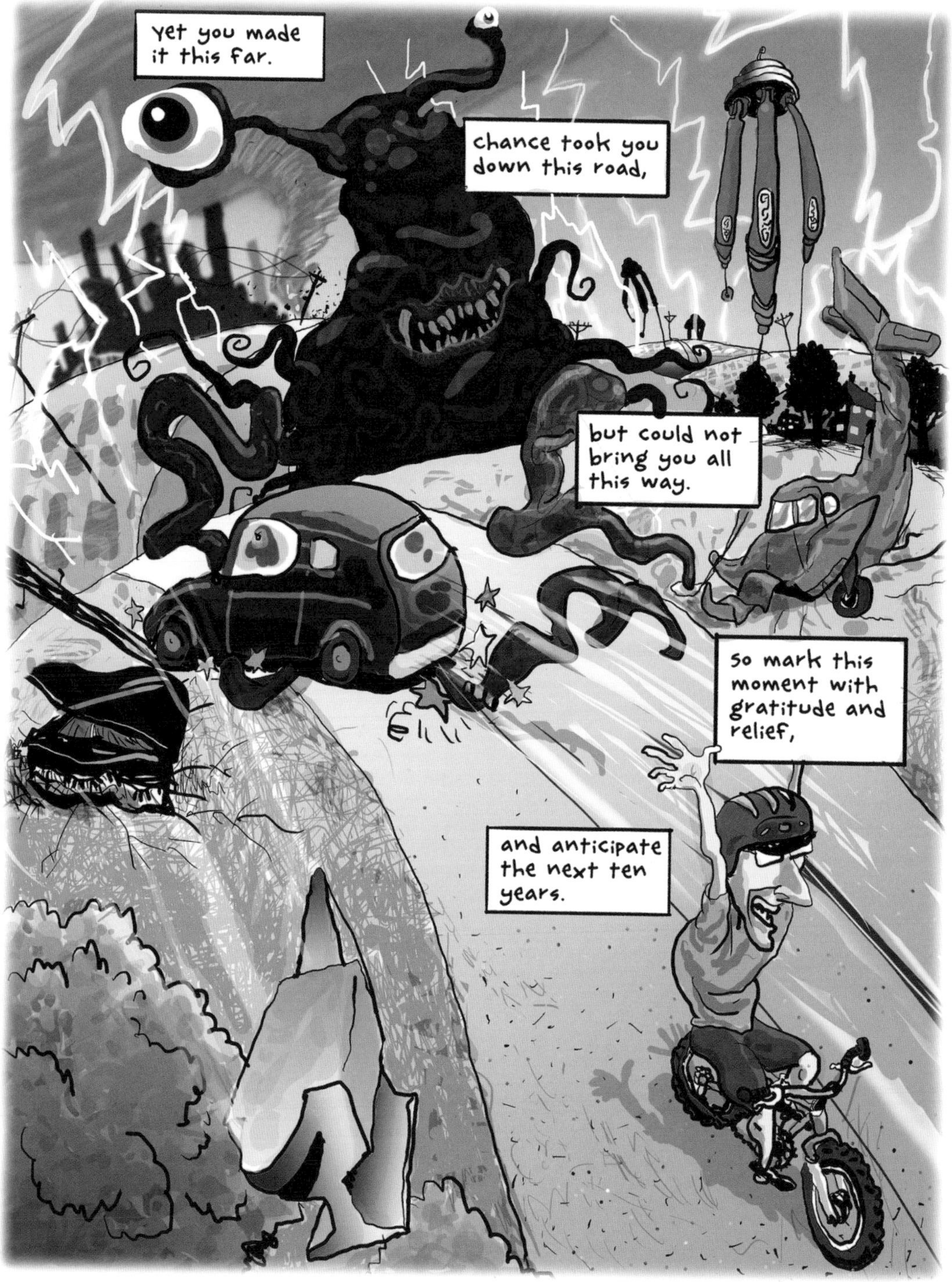
yet you made it this far.
chance took you down this road,
but could not bring you all this way.
so mark this moment with gratitude and relief,
and anticipate the next ten years.